Contents

Acknowledgements

First edition

All books are team efforts and this one is no exception. Although it is impossible to name everyone who has contributed to the preparation of this book, we should like to acknowledge our particular debt to the following people. People with Parkinson's and others provided a wide-ranging selection of questions. We are particularly grateful to all the people with Parkinson's and their families, from whom we have learned – and continue to learn – so much, and would like to dedicate this book to them.

- Members of YAPP&RS for responding to requests for questions and their chairman Keith Levett for reading the manuscript.
- Bridget McCall (Information Manager) at the Parkinson's Disease Society for prompt practical assistance in retrieving information, patient reading of drafts and redrafts, and unstinting moral support and encouragement.
- Franklin MacDonald (Welfare and Benefits Adviser), Anne Mathon (Counsellor) and other staff members at the Parkinson's Disease Society for relevant questions and much specialist information and advice.
- Jane Stewart (Nurse Specialist) for specialist information on apomorphine and Parkinson's Nurse Specialists.
- Doctors Lloyd A. Frost, Hardev Pall and Andrew Lees for reading the manuscript and making helpful comments and suggestions.

- Linda Moore, our cartoonist, for being the only member of the team to meet her deadlines and for inspiring us with her perceptive and humorous cartoons.
- Les and Lilla Pickford for agreeing to be photographed so that our commitment to reality could extend to the book's cover.

Second edition

In working on this first full revision, we have appreciated the generous help of the following Parkinson's Disease Society staff:

- Bridget McCall (Information Manager)
- Mary Baker (Chief Executive)
- Helen Barber (Information Officer)
- John Bucknall (Welfare Benefits and Employment Rights Adviser)
- Rosie Hayward (Placements Adviser)
- Barbara Cormie (Publications Manager)

We were saddened by the deaths in 1998 of Professor David Marsden and Les Pickford, who in different ways made major contributions to our first edition and we offer our condolences to their families.

Lastly we welcome our new cover team, Leo Cunningham, Vina Curren and Michael Harmsworth, all of whom have Parkinson's and so represent the special people for whom this book is written.

Third edition

Dr Marie Oxtoby who was the original co-author of this book has decided to step down and has passed her mantle onto Bridget McCall, Information Manager at the Parkinson's Disease Society of the United Kingdom. We hope that the 3rd edition continues to reflect Marie's considerable wisdom and insight into the needs of all of you who read this book and are living with Parkinson's.

Bridget McCall would like to thank the following people who have contributed advice, information and support during the development of the 3rd edition of *Parkinson's – the 'at your fingertips' guide.*

- Angela Birleson, Occupational Therapist
- John Bucknall, PDS Welfare and Employment Rights Manager
- Frances Carroll, previously PDS staff member
- Barbara Cormie, PDS Publications Manager
- Colin Cosgrove, PDS Information Officer
- Wendy Darch, previously PDS staff member
- Caroline Evans, Parkinson's Disease Nurse Specialist
- Alison Forbes, Parkinson's Disease Nurse Specialist
- Dr Duncan Forsyth, Consultant Geriatrician
- Kirstin Goldring, PDS Brain Tissue Bank
- Rosie Hayward, PDS Development Worker
- Calvin Johnson, Medical Information and Drug Safety Executive, Britannia Pharmaceuticals Ltd
- Anna Jones, Physiotherapist
- Sue Lester, PDS Information and Publications Assistant
- Dr Tony Luxton, Consultant Geriatrician
- James Motley, previously at Britannia Pharmaceuticals
- Lynne Osborne, Parkinson's Disease Nurse Specialist
- Bhanu Ramaswamy, Physiotherapist
- Ruth Reed, PDS Helpline nurse
- Sheila Scott, Speech and Language Therapist and PDS Education Manager
- Professor Terry Stacey, Director of COREC
- Helen Weldon, PDS Development Worker

Foreword

by Linda Kelly
Chief Executive of the Parkinson's Disease Society

When you first hear the news that you, a family member or a close friend has Parkinson's, the effect can be devastating. What is it? Can it be cured? What can I do? Why me? These are just a few of the questions that need answering.

Parkinson's – the 'at your fingertips' guide aims to provide simple, clear answers to the many questions that people with Parkinson's, their carers and families face not only at diagnosis but throughout their lives. This book gathers the experiences of many people facing these issues themselves and tries to help and support people living with Parkinson's today.

I hope it will help and assist you.

Linda Kelly

Introduction

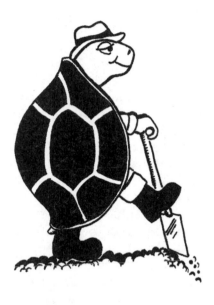

If you are someone who has Parkinson's, or if you have a relative or friend with Parkinson's, then this book is intended for you. Its starting point is the important questions which you and people like you ask every day. The questions are real questions that we have been asked by real people and, in answering them clearly and honestly, we hope to improve your access to information and help so that you can get on with your life as normally as possible.

We believe that, if you are well informed and involved in decisions about your own care, your treatment will be more successful and you will feel more in control. We also hope that the information in this book will be of interest to the doctors, nurses, therapists and other professionals who work with people like you, and will help them to be more aware of the everyday implications of living with Parkinson's.

1

Parkinson's is an extremely complicated and variable condition. People can and do live with it for 20 years and more. Being diagnosed does not mean that someone's symptoms will get worse – in fact, the reverse is more likely to be true. Although there is as yet no cure, there are some effective treatments and more are being developed.

No two people are exactly alike either in their symptoms or in their response to treatment, so the questions and answers in this book cover a vast range of situations from the most mild to the most serious. It is impossible for anyone to suggest any one treatment or course of action which would be right for everyone, and we have not tried to do so. Instead we have tried to provide you with information about the various options that are available, as well as the organizations or people to whom you can turn for more detailed personal help and advice.

This includes the Parkinson's Disease Society of the United Kingdom (PDS), which is the main source of information and support on Parkinson's in the UK. If the PDS has a particular information resource on a subject under discussion in the text, this has been indicated. Details of the work of the PDS and how to obtain these resources is contained in Chapter 15.

The medical condition with which we are concerned in this book is Parkinson's disease, named after Dr James Parkinson, a remarkable and talented London doctor who, in 1817, first properly described its main features and outlined the course of the illness. However, you will notice that we refer throughout to *Parkinson's* rather than *Parkinson's disease*. This is because we know from experience that many people are distressed by the word 'disease' and would find its constant repetition distracting and upsetting. Although the medical textbooks are unlikely to change, many voluntary organizations around the world now use this shortened name. It is certainly easier to say and this book will also be several pages shorter as a result of our decision!

Neurology, the branch of medicine involved with Parkinson's, uses many very technical terms to refer to the complex range of symptoms and side effects. We have used, and explained, those terms which are in most frequent use (there is also a glossary at the back of the book for easy reference) but otherwise we have tried to avoid technical language and jargon. Words that appear in the **Glossary** are in *italic* on first mention in the text.

Drug names are also confusing – and subject to change. Most drugs have at least two names, the generic or true name and the trade (or brand) name given by the company that makes the drug. Usually we give both versions, using small first letters for the generic name and capital first letters for the trade name.

Parkinson's – the 'at your fingertips' guide may strike some people as a rather odd title, as one of the symptoms of Parkinson's is that it can make fine movements of the fingers more difficult. The reason for the title is that the book belongs to a series of books about different conditions, all of which are intended to provide accessible and reader-friendly information (you will find details of other books in the series at the back of this book). We hope that we have succeeded in this aim! Evidence that people with Parkinson's can use their fingers very effectively is provided by our cartoonist, Linda Moore, a younger person with Parkinson's who works as a teacher and leads a very active life. We hope that you like her drawings as much as we do, and that you will be encouraged by her constructive and sometimes humorous approach to Parkinson's. She chose the tortoise as her 'character' because slowness is an important feature of the condition but also because, as the fables remind us, tortoises always get there in the end!

How to use this book

The book is not intended to be read from cover to cover but to be used selectively to meet your own particular situation. It has a detailed list of contents and a comprehensive index so that you can quickly identify the parts which are relevant to you. For example, people who are newly diagnosed might want to find out more about the nature of Parkinson's (in Chapter 1), its main symptoms (in Chapter 2) and the treatment that they have been given (in Chapter 3). They may also want to look at Chapters 4 and 5 which address questions of access to treatment and of attitudes and relationships. People still at work might want to concentrate on the appropriate section of Chapter 8, and may find some of the financial information in Chapter 12 useful. The carers of people with advanced Parkinson's will find helpful information about support for carers in Chapter 6, advice on benefits in Chapter 12, and discussion of options for care outside the home in Chapter 13. Chapter 14 has been fully revised. Numerous information sheets and booklets from the PDS are mentioned throughout the text – see Appendix 1 for their address and Appendix 2 for details about their publications.

Please remember that a book like this cannot provide exact and full answers to your individual problems. What it can do is to provide you with the information which will help you to obtain those answers from doctors, health professionals and workers in the voluntary and statutory services in your own area.

Not everyone will agree with the answers we give, but future editions of this book can only be improved if you let us know when you disagree and have found our advice to be unhelpful. We would also like to know if there are important questions that we have not covered. Please write to us c/o Class Publishing, Barb House, Barb Mews, London W6 7PA.

1
What is Parkinson's?

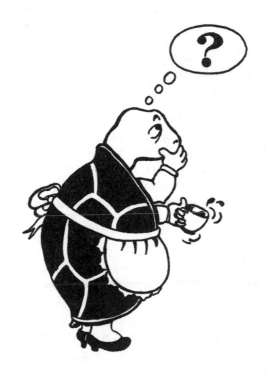

This chapter tries to address some difficult questions about the nature of Parkinson's – difficult because we do not yet know all the answers. We have tried to be honest where this is the case and those interested in research developments can turn to Chapter 14 where the continuing search for answers is discussed further.

What is Parkinson's disease

Parkinson's is a progressive neurological condition with three main symptoms:

- *Tremor* – which usually begins in one hand or arm and is more likely to occur when the affected part of the body is at rest and decrease when it is being used. Stress can make the tremor more noticeable. However the presence of tremor does not necessarily mean a that person has Parkinson's, as there are several other types and causes of tremor. Also, although most people associate Parkinson's with tremor, up to 30% of people with Parkinson's do not have this symptom.

- Slowness of movement (*bradykinesia*) and stiffness of muscles (*rigidity*) – movements can become difficult to initiate, take longer to perform and lack coordination. People with Parkinson's often have problems with turning round, getting out of a chair, rolling over in bed, stooped posture, and making fine finger movements, facial expressions and body language.

Other symptoms can include tiredness, depression, and difficulties with handwriting, speech and balance.

The symptoms usually begin slowly, develop gradually, and in no particular order. Parkinson's is a very individual condition and each person will have a different collection of symptoms and response to treatment. The rate at which the condition progresses, the nature and severity of symptoms is also individual.

What is parkinsonism and how does differ from Parkinson's disease?

The main symptoms of Parkinson's (tremor, stiffness and slowness of movement) are also the main symptoms of a collective group of conditions known as parkinsonism. Parkinson's is the most common form of parkinsonism and is sometimes referred to as idiopathic Parkinson's disease, which means its cause is unknown. Less common forms of parkinsonism include multiple system atrophy (MSA), progressive supranuclear palsy (PSP) and drug-induced parkinsonism. The PDS (Parkinson's Disease Society – see Chapter 15) has an information sheet on *Parkinsonism* (FS14) which provides more information.

The cause – or causes – of Parkinson's

What goes wrong in Parkinson's?

In Parkinson's, a small part of the brain called the *substantia nigra* (see Figure 1.1) loses a lot of its nerve cells and so is unable to function normally. These nerve cells use a chemical known as *dopamine* to send messages to other parts of the brain and spinal

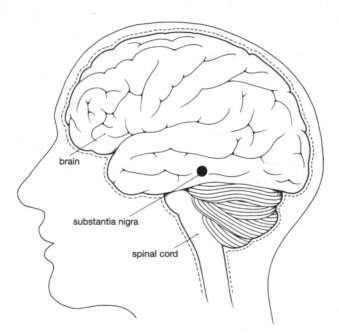

Figure 1.1 Location of the substantia nigra

cord that control coordination of movement. The substantia nigra has been described as the gearbox of the brain. When it stops working properly it leads to tremors (shaking), over-rigidity of the muscles (stiffness), slowness and uncoordinated movement. These effects often show up as difficulties with arm and leg movements or, less often, as problems with speech. Remember, though, that they will not all affect every person with Parkinson's. They often start on one side of the body and, although there is a general tendency for them to spread to the other side, they can sometimes remain on just the one side for many years.

What causes the brain to stop making dopamine?

Dopamine is made by the cells in the substantia nigra. Brain cells die all the time but, in Parkinson's, these particular cells die earlier than they should. We do not need all the cells to continue functioning normally, and it is estimated that about 70% of the cells in the substantia nigra have to be lost before the symptoms of Parkinson's begin to show. After this point the remaining cells cannot produce enough dopamine to keep the body's motor system running smoothly. The question which research is still trying to answer is why these cells die. Possibilities include genetic predisposition to viruses, poisons in the environment and shortages of protective chemicals in the brain.

My father's Parkinson's appeared after he had had a bad accident at work and I have met other people with similar experiences, so can shocks cause Parkinson's?

We know that by the time the first symptoms of Parkinson's appear, many of the cells in the substantia nigra have already died, so most researchers believe that the disease process has been happening unnoticed for at least five years. It is therefore unlikely that any shock (such as your father's accident) that happened immediately before the symptoms appeared has played much part in causing Parkinson's. However, a period of anxiety or *depression* could possibly bring on symptoms that otherwise would have appeared weeks or months later. This is easiest to understand in the case of tremor. We all have some tremor and, if we are anxious, it will show. So, if someone who is on the threshold of developing the tremor of Parkinson's gets upset, it is easy to see how this could become noticeable earlier.

I saw the word 'idiopathic' written before Parkinson's in my husband's medical notes. What does it mean?

The word *idiopathic* simply means that the cause is not known. This is true for everyone with Parkinson's except those in whom it is caused by drugs or (very rarely) by *encephalitis lethargica*, or when it is clearly genetic, so it is hardly necessary to use the term at all. Not knowing the cause of a disease is common and one could equally well use the term 'idiopathic' in front of diabetes or high blood pressure or many other illnesses. Drug-induced parkinsonism is discussed in the answer to the next question, and there is more information about encephalitis lethargica and genetic causes later in this chapter.

What is drug-induced Parkinson's?

As the name implies, this is a form of parkinsonism, which is caused by taking certain drugs. The drugs involved are mainly those used for serious psychiatric problems, known as neuroleptics, not the ones normally used to relieve anxiety or depression. Other drugs can also cause drug-induced parkinsonism, such as prochlorperazine (Stemetil), which is used to control dizziness, or metoclopramide (Maxolon), which is prescribed for nausea. The PDS has an information sheet on *Drug-induced Parkinsonism* (FS38) which gives details of others and general information on managing this condition.

By coincidence, some people with real Parkinson's may have taken some of these drugs for a short period. The difference is that, in cases caused by these drugs, the symptoms will wear off over a few weeks or months once the drug has been stopped.

There is another, rare, sense in which the phrase 'drug-induced Parkinson's' is used – a substance known as MPTP taken by some American drug addicts in the early 1980s caused symptoms almost identical to those seen in Parkinson's. There is more information about this in Chapter 14 on **Research and clinical trials**.

I hate the word 'disease' and felt very upset when given the diagnosis – it sounds like something infectious or catching. Is it?

Parkinson's is certainly not catching or infectious. At the moment, even a virus seems an unlikely cause for Parkinson's but, even if it were later shown to be a cause, it is inconceivable that it would be infectious to others.

'Disease' can sound a rather harsh word, especially as there are many more serious conditions that do not carry this label. The official title is unlikely to be changed, although many people in the UK and around the world are now referring to the condition as Parkinson's or PD. Use the description that you find most acceptable and try to develop a positive attitude towards your condition. We know this can help, and we discuss it in more detail in Chapter 5 on **Attitudes and relationships**.

Who gets Parkinson's?

I know that they say Parkinson's is not hereditary but I have it and so do two of my cousins. How can the doctors be sure?

Researchers have looked carefully at people with Parkinson's and at their families and, in most cases, there is no other member of the family with the condition. Certainly the illness is only rarely hereditary in the usual sense of the term, in that neither the mother, father, brothers or sisters have had the illness. Someone who has been diagnosed need have no worries about their own children or siblings even if they are identical twins.

Having said that, if one looks in the wider family, for example cousins (as in your case), there is a slightly higher frequency of the illness than one would expect by chance. There are also very rare examples where one cannot doubt that Parkinson's is in the family. These rare families are of great interest to researchers and, very recently, genetic mutations have been described in *genes* found within these families, and specific *proteins* produced by the genes have been identified.

However, there are also cases in which everyone believes that there are several family members with Parkinson's but, on closer examination, it turns out that family members with a *familial tremor* (see Chapter 2 for more information about this) are being counted as if they had Parkinson's.

Does Parkinson's have a genetic component even though it is not hereditary?

Another way of putting this question might be: 'Does Parkinson's have something to do with a person's genes (the building blocks controlling the amount and type of proteins produced), which then affects various interactions with each other and environmental factors, even though it is not handed down directly from parent to child?' This is an important question, but it is impossible to give a simple answer.

Researchers went through a stage of thinking that the genetic component in Parkinson's was very small because it was very rare for both members of a set of twins to get the illness. However, this was true both of identical and non-identical twins. To really test whether or not there is a genetic component, one needs to see a difference between the two types of twins. As an example, if there was a strong genetic component, both members of sets of identical twins would get the illness much more frequently than non-identical twins. The numbers of twins found and tested was initially insufficient to come to a definite conclusion, but recent work suggests a considerable genetic component in people who develop Parkinson's under the age of 50, and little or no genetic influence in those who develop it later.

Most people now believe that, as with many other common conditions, Parkinson's is likely to have a genetic component which makes some individuals susceptible to something in the environment, perhaps a chemical or a virus. Intriguing though this is, it does not alter the fact that the risk of the children of people with Parkinson's also developing the condition is negligible.

Is Parkinson's more common in men than in women?

At each age Parkinson's is somewhat more common in men than in women. Some studies have suggested that men are twice as likely to get it. However, as women on the whole live longer than men, and as the disease gets commoner with age, there are just as many women as men alive with Parkinson's.

I read somewhere that Parkinson's is found all over the world. Is this true or is it more common in some countries or climates?

Yes, Parkinson's is found worldwide. We do not always know what the exact figures are, as good research counting the number of people with Parkinson's is not available from every country. From what we do know, it does appear that Parkinson's is possibly less common in countries closer to the equator than it is in the UK.

My sister is 37 and has been having trouble with her walking for some time. We thought it was a trapped nerve but now the doctor says it is Parkinson's. I can't believe it – surely Parkinson's is an old person's disease?

At 37 your sister is certainly young to get Parkinson's, but it is by no means unheard of at that age. Michael J. Fox, the Canadian TV and film actor was only 30 when he was diagnosed and all neurologists will have seen people with Parkinson's in their thirties and even younger. The illness is certainly much more common in elderly people but can affect those in relative youth. It is estimated that 1 in 20 of those diagnosed are under the age of 40.

You will find many references throughout this book to the special problems and needs of younger people with Parkinson's and to a self-help group, the YAPP&Rs, which brings them together and offers valuable support and encouragement. YAPP&Rs is a special interest group of the PDS and you will find more information about their activities in Chapter 14. The PDS also has an information pack for younger people with Parkinson's called *One in Twenty* (B77), which provides information on young-onset Parkinson's and contributions from other younger people with Parkinson's about how they cope.

Recently we visited an old friend who has been told she has Parkinson's. She keeps asking herself 'Why me?' and wondering if there is anything she could have done to cause it. We reassured her that it was not her fault. Were we right to do so?

You were quite right to reassure her. It is natural to want an explanation for an illness and common for some people, particularly if they are a bit depressed, to be tempted to blame themselves. Bad habits certainly do not cause Parkinson's! Although we cannot yet answer the 'Why me?' question, nobody believes that the cause or causes of Parkinson's will turn out to be something under the control of those who get it. If your friend continues to blame herself, it would be worth you and her doctor considering whether or not she is depressed.

I am 68 and have always looked after myself. I do not smoke or drink to excess but now I am having all kinds of difficulties and the doctors have diagnosed Parkinson's. Why me?

As stated elsewhere in this book, the cause of Parkinson's is unknown and 'Why me?' is the crucial question for researchers to answer. Alcohol does not appear to be involved to any extent and the question of smoking is uncertain (see the answer to the next question). You are too young to have been involved in the epidemics of *sleeping sickness* (encephalitis lethargica) that were around at the time of World War I and which caused a special kind of Parkinson's. There has recently been some evidence that the body's inherited ability to turn harmful chemicals into harmless substances may be somewhat reduced in people who get Parkinson's, but this is an area for future research rather than an established fact at present.

Is it true that smoking cigarettes can protect people from Parkinson's?

Most research surveys have suggested that people who get Parkinson's have on the whole smoked remarkably little. One difficulty of these surveys is that they are biased because some smokers who should really have been included in the survey have already died of other causes, such as cancer. It is also possible that, before symptoms become obvious, there is something that makes individuals who are destined to get Parkinson's just not enjoy smoking. It remains a possibility that smoking genuinely protects people from getting Parkinson's. One day we will be able to protect people from getting Parkinson's but smoking (which causes so much death and disability) will not be a part of the answer!

Outlook

Is there a cure for Parkinson's?

No, there is no cure yet. Most medical success stories are due to prevention rather than cure, and this is particularly likely in *neurological conditions* (conditions affecting the body's nervous system), such as Parkinson's, that are linked to the loss of nerve cells. To prevent something happening, we need to understand its cause, so research into the cause or causes of Parkinson's has to continue (see Chapter 14 on *Research and clinical trials* for more information about this). Meanwhile, there are treatments available (they are discussed in Chapter 3), so the overall situation is more favourable then in many other neurological conditions. The discovery of a way of slowing down the already fairly slow progression of Parkinson's would be a real step forward. To date, we have seen some false dawns, but there is still intense interest among researchers in identifying drugs that may protect against further cell death.

Will I die from Parkinson's?

Parkinson's by itself does not directly cause people to die. Life expectancy with good treatment is not much changed from normal life expectancy, and none of the drugs that are used for Parkinson's have any serious *side effects* that could cause death. However, in people who are seriously disabled (usually those who have had Parkinson's for many years), their general physical and mental condition can either cause or exacerbate other illnesses and so contribute to the final cause of death. Examples would include a greater risk of falls leading to fractures and a higher risk of infections like pneumonia.

I have a tremor in one hand. Will it spread? Should I learn to write with my other hand?

As with other aspects of Parkinson's, tremor is a slowly progressive problem and, in the end, symptoms are likely to worsen and spread to the other side of your body. Parkinson's is very variable, so some people who start with tremor in one hand live for many years before it spreads to the other side, whilst in other people this happens more quickly. In a lucky few it stays on the one side.

Because of this unpredictability, it is difficult for us to answer the second part of your question. The possible long-term advantages of learning to use your other hand have to be weighed against the certainty that using your non-dominant side will make writing and other activities more difficult now. You might also find such efforts stressful, which could have an effect on your tremor (there is a question about the effects of stress in Chapter 2).

If handwriting is a particular problem for you, we would suggest you contact an occupational therapist for advice. See the physical therapies section of Chapter 2 for more information on their role and how to access them. The PDS also has an information sheet on *Handwriting* (FS23).

My brother, aged 48, was told he had Parkinson's a year ago. How quickly does it progress and could he end up in a wheelchair?

Most people with Parkinson's respond either well or very well to treatment, particularly when, as in your brother's case, it comes on at a fairly early age. You are probably going to see an improvement with treatment (rather than a deterioration) for several years to come. However, underneath this improvement, the dopamine nerve cells are gradually dying and eventually his response to treatment will tend to be less good. This may not become a problem for some five to 10 years.

The permanent use of a wheelchair is not common in Parkinson's. Although we cannot say for sure that your brother will never need to use a wheelchair, he is likely to be a good 20 years off any likelihood of needing one. Remember too that a wheelchair can extend, rather than limit, people's horizons – we discuss the practical aspects of mobility in Chapter 11 on *Getting around on wheels*.

2
Symptoms and diagnosis

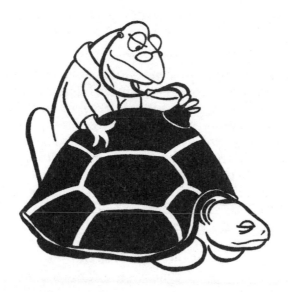

No two people with Parkinson's are the same, and the initial symptoms in the first few years can vary markedly between different individuals. As time goes by, the differences in the way it affects people become even more noticeable, and certain symptoms and complications of treatment will simply **never** occur in many individuals. We also have to remember the effects of ageing – as people get older, some of the symptoms attributed to Parkinson's may really be caused by the ageing process itself, or by some other illness. This is particularly true of symptoms such as bladder problems, memory disorders, confusion, and aches and pains, where Parkinson's may be only one of several factors involved.

It is therefore very important that, as you read or dip into this chapter, you do not assume that you or your relatives will experience every symptom that is mentioned.

Problems of diagnosis

My Parkinson's was diagnosed four years ago but I was attending my doctor for two years before that. Is it difficult to diagnose?

The diagnosis of Parkinson's can be difficult and it is very common for people to realize, after the diagnosis has been made, that the symptoms have been there for longer than was first thought. These earlier symptoms could have led to your visits to the doctor, especially as some of them are rather vague and easily attributable to getting older, or to being a bit depressed, or they may have an arthritic flavour to them. The cause of a tremor can be difficult to diagnose as there is a common variety of tremor known as familial or essential tremor (see the next question for more information about this) which can be confused with Parkinson's.

As there is no laboratory test for Parkinson's, a doctor may not be able to be sure about the diagnosis until time passes and a change in the overall picture makes the Parkinson's more obvious or rules it out. Most doctors will not want to say it is Parkinson's until they are sure. This will usually be when at least two of the three main symptoms (tremor, slowness of movement and stiffness) are present.

What are the other medical conditions that sometimes get confused with Parkinson's?

There are several conditions that may need to be considered by your doctors.

- *Essential tremor* (otherwise known as familial or *senile tremor*) is a common cause of diagnostic confusion.

Usually an essential tremor has been there, even if in a milder form, for many years and, in over half the cases, there is known to be a tremor in the family. By contrast, finding another member of the family with Parkinson's is rare. An essential tremor becomes worse with anxiety and rather better with small amounts of alcohol. Essential tremor is at its worst with the arms outstretched or when you are holding a cup of tea or writing, whereas the tremor of Parkinson's is usually most obvious when the arm is doing nothing and at rest (which is why it is sometimes described as a *resting tremor*). The tremor of Parkinson's is also quite often on one side. However, there are exceptions that make diagnosis difficult, particularly when the tremor appears to have come on recently but looks like an essential tremor. It is at this stage that the diagnostic skills of a specialist can be helpful, but a totally confident diagnosis may still not be possible at the first consultation. The Tremor Foundation can provide information support on essential tremor (see Appendix 1 for contact details)

- A shuffling gait (looking rather like the one sometimes seen in Parkinson's) can occur in elderly people who are known to have had a stroke or high blood pressure. It is caused by hardening of the arteries rather than by Parkinson's. In such cases other symptoms that are often found in Parkinson's (such as tremor, stiffness and lack of coordination of movements other than walking) are usually absent.

- Some drugs can cause side effects that resemble Parkinson's. However, this form of Parkinson's will get better when the drugs are stopped, although the improvement may take many months. (There is a question about drug-induced Parkinson's in Chapter 1.) See the PDS information sheet on *Drug-induced Parkinsonism* (FS38) for more information.

- There are some rare conditions which begin by looking like Parkinson's but which then turn out to be untypical and which are harder to treat. These include multiple system atrophy (MSA), progressive supranuclear palsy (PSP) and cortical basal degeneration (CBD). The PDS helps people with these conditions. In addition, the Sarah Matheson Trust supports people with MSA, and the Progressive Supranuclear Palsy (Europe) Association supports people with PSP and CBD. All these organizations also support research into these conditions (see Appendix 1 for contact details). See the PDS information sheet on *Parkinsonism* (FS14) for more information.

I know Parkinson's is something to do with the brain and I thought the doctor at the hospital would send me for a brain scan but she didn't. Why not?

The substantia nigra (the part of the brain affected in Parkinson's) is very small and cannot be seen on the type of brain scans that are available at the moment. The two usual types of scan, *CT* and *MRI*, look normal in someone with Parkinson's. Such scans are therefore only used when the doctor has a serious worry that it could be another condition such as a brain tumour, a blockage of the system that drains the fluid in the brain, or a stroke. As these concerns are rare, for most people a brain scan is not necessary.

Two other kinds of scan, *PET (Positron Emission Tomography)* and *SPECT (Single Photon Emission Computed Tomography)*, which use radioactive labels, are currently being used by researchers, and can show the loss of dopamine activity, characteristic of Parkinson's but which can also be caused by other types of parkinsonism. However, PET and SPECT cannot be reliably used to differentiate the different types of parkinsonism from each other. The SPECT scan, also called DaTSCAN, has been developed and is usually used to separate essential tremor (see previous question) from other kinds of tremulous parkinsonism, in the few cases where the diagnosis cannot be made using clinical observation and medical history alone.

My friend has recently been told he has Parkinson's and he was sent up to a special clinic in London to have his tremor measured. What good will that do?

Your friend has probably been asked to go to the clinic as part of a research study to measure his tremor more accurately than a doctor can do in an ordinary clinic. Such careful measurements contribute to our understanding of Parkinson's and other neurological conditions, but they are not necessary for the diagnosis of Parkinson's. Your friend may, however, derive overall benefit from seeing doctors with a special interest in Parkinson's.

What should I do? My doctor says that I have Parkinson's but my friends don't believe it and really I don't either.

All doctors accept that their patients could be correct in this situation, particularly when there is no special test. The thing to do would be to go back to your GP and ask him or her how sure they are about the diagnosis. Parkinson's can usually be diagnosed only with reasonable certainty when two of the three main symptoms are present (see the next question for more information about them). If it is a problem of tremor with no other symptoms or physical signs, your GP may accept that the diagnosis cannot be substantiated with confidence. By the end of the discussion you may both have decided that it would be worthwhile to get the opinion of a specialist. If you have already seen a specialist and still do not believe or accept the diagnosis, you could ask for a second opinion. If your GP and one or two specialists all agree that it is Parkinson's, you should probably accept that your friends might be wrong! An alternative is to press for a DaTSCAN.

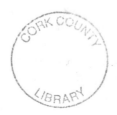

The main symptoms

An aunt in America has just written to say she has Parkinson's. I gather it is a complex condition and varies a lot between people, but what are the main symptoms?

You are quite right in saying that symptoms vary a lot between people. There are three main symptoms of Parkinson's – tremor, slowness and rigidity.

- **Tremor**, often mainly on one side, often in a hand or arm is a common early symptom. It is most obvious when the affected part of the body is at rest and will often decrease or disappear when the part is in use. Tremor may also come and go and often becomes more noticeable when the person with Parkinson's is anxious or excited. About half of the people with Parkinson's start off with a tremor and, although often obvious and embarrassing (because it happens when the hand is at rest), it is not as much of a problem as might be thought at first glance. About 70% of people with Parkinson's have a tremor and it is slightly less common in younger people with Parkinson's.

- Slowness of movement (**bradykinesia**) and lack of coordination is another sign of Parkinson's and creates more problems for people than the better-known tremor. Slowness can also be mainly on one side. Tasks take longer and require more concentration instead of being done automatically and without thinking. Difficulty with doing up buttons, brushing teeth or shaving are common ways in which the problem comes to light. Handwriting can be affected, becoming more difficult, smaller and less legible. The technical name for the type of smaller writing found in Parkinson's is *micrographia*. The arm may not swing normally whilst walking and this is a sign that the specialist often looks for carefully. A tendency to shuffle and to walk slowly is a common way for Parkinson's to appear, although falling is rarely a feature in the first stages. Facial expression often becomes less animated (the so-called '*poker*' or '*mask*' *face*) and speech may become slower and more monotonous, though it usually remains comprehensible.

- Stiffness of the muscles (**rigidity**) is the other major symptom.

Other symptoms can include tiredness, depression, difficulties with communication (including speech and facial expression), and balance problems.

My father, who has come to live with us, has Parkinson's. I think he is settling down but he does not look very happy and hardly ever smiles. Is this the Parkinson's too?

Almost certainly. Lack of facial expression is a feature of Parkinson's (as mentioned in the previous answer) and is often noticed first by relatives, particularly husbands or wives. While it can be helpful to the specialist in making a diagnosis, it is a distressing feature of the condition for the people themselves and for their relatives and can lead to much misunderstanding. We have discussed this important topic further in Chapter 5 and 7. Speech and language therapists can advise on ways of overcoming problems with facial expression. See the *Physical therapies* section of Chapter 3 for more information on the role of speech and language therapy in Parkinson's. The PDS also has information on all aspects of communication and Parkinson's.

I used to be proud of my handwriting and won prizes at school. Now it is small and spidery. Can I blame Parkinson's for this?

Writing is often affected by Parkinson's. Characteristically it does get smaller (micrographia), and so you can probably blame your Parkinson's for the change in your handwriting. There are other causes of handwriting problems although they rarely have the effect of making the writing smaller. For example, very trembly writing is usually caused by a form of essential tremor rather than by Parkinson's. Difficulty with writing which is unaccompanied by other problems is usually caused by writer's cramp, which is a form of *dystonia*. (There is more information about essential tremor in the previous section of this chapter on **Problems of diagnosis** and more about dystonia in the next section on **Other possible symptoms**.)

An occupational therapist can advise on ways of overcoming problems with handwriting (see the **Physical therapies** section of Chapter 3 for more information on their role in Parkinson's). The PDS has an information sheet on *Handwriting* (FS23).

I love walking but now my feet do not always cooperate. How does Parkinson's interfere with walking?

Before we actually answer your question, we would like to stress how important it is for you to try and carry on walking, particularly as you like it so much. Keeping active, both mentally and physically, is a very important way of dealing with Parkinson's. You might find that having a companion with you on your walks or simply using a walking stick will give you extra confidence and there are further suggestions in Chapter 9 which could help.

Parkinson's can certainly affect walking in a number of ways through the combined effects of slowness and rigidity. As with most of the other features of Parkinson's, it varies enormously between individuals and usually responds well to medication, especially in the early years.

The mildest way in which Parkinson's affects walking is through the loss of arm swing on either one or both sides, something which does not have any serious ill effects. In time the walking can slow down and there is a tendency to hunch the shoulders; later it may develop into a shuffling, somewhat unsteady gait. At a more advanced stage, there may be particular difficulties with cornering, starting off and stopping, or going through doorways.

A physiotherapist can advise on ways of overcoming problems with walking. See the **Physical therapies** section of Chapter 3 for further information on their role in Parkinson's. The PDS has an information sheet on *Physiotherapy* (FS42).

Sometimes when walking I stop suddenly and my feet seem to be stuck to the floor. I think it is called 'freezing'. What makes it happen?

You are quite right that this is known as *freezing*. Nobody understands quite why it happens. Sometimes it is triggered by being anxious or in an unfamiliar or crowded place. Approaching a doorway or negotiating confined spaces can create special problems, but at other times it can occur out of the blue. There are ways of trying to overcome it, which we will discuss in Chapter 3 on *Treatment* and Chapter 9 on *Managing at home*. The PDS has an information sheet on *Freezing* (FS63).

I know that lack of balance and falling are fairly common among people with Parkinson's. Why should this be?

Loss of balance and falling are indeed features of Parkinson's, because the part of the brain that is affected by Parkinson's is one of the areas which is important for balance. However, such problems are very rare in the early years, nor do they happen to everybody, however long they have had the illness. Chapter 9 on *Managing at home* gives some ideas that may help you overcome the problem. The PDS has an information sheet on *Falls* (FS39).

My husband's voice has become quite quiet but, more upsetting for me, is the loss of colour and expression. Is this a common feature of Parkinson's?

Some people with Parkinson's do get problems with their voices. It is rarely the first feature to be noticed and more often develops later when other parts of the body are more seriously affected. However, what you have noticed is not uncommon – that is that the voice becomes quiet and monotonous. The loss of colour and expression is upsetting for both the person with Parkinson's and for those who are close to them. There is often, but not always, a good response to drug treatment. Speech therapy can help improve communication. Chapter 7 on *Communication* contains more information.

I take my tablets and get around fairly well but I get dreadfully tired and often cannot do the things I want. Why should this be?

Tiredness can be a feature of Parkinson's, particularly if your response to treatment has not been very good. The extra effort needed for actions that used to be spontaneous can be exhausting. It may be worth asking your GP or specialist whether you are taking as much medication as is desirable, or whether it would be worth taking more, at least for a trial period. It is also possible that your tiredness is due to depression. Depression is an odd word often used differently by the man or woman in the street and by doctors. Sometimes people who would be diagnosed by doctors as depressed (and so considered for *antidepressant* medication) do not think of themselves as depressed. Rather they complain of being tired all the time, or of the response to their treatment being less good than they expected. There is a question at the beginning of the next section about depression in Parkinson's. The PDS has an information sheet on *Fatigue* (FS72).

Are the symptoms likely to be worse when I am feeling under stress?

Very much so. In Parkinson's, as in many aspects of life, stress is unhelpful: the more you are stressed, the worse your symptoms will appear to be. And just as anyone can tremble if they are very stressed, so stress is likely to exaggerate any tremor from your Parkinson's.

It is actually quite difficult for any of us to recognize when we are under stress. There may be occasions when your doctor thinks some of your symptoms are related to stress, even though you yourself do not feel particularly stressed at that time.

Many people who are under stress also sleep badly. Sleep is important in Parkinson's and, like most other people, you will probably feel better after a good rest. Keeping active and learning how to relax are important but, if you have serious problems with sleeping, you should consult your doctor.

Other possible symptoms

How common is depression in people with Parkinson's?

Depression is common, and most people with Parkinson's will have some degree of it at one time or another. It can happen at any stage and indeed occasionally appears before the physical symptoms. For this reason it is generally believed to be part of the illness and not only a reaction to it – the chemical changes in the brain (that are connected with the Parkinson's) may lead to a biochemical form of depression. On the other hand any kind of illness, even a relatively mild one, can make people feel depressed and nearly everyone with Parkinson's will have their moments of low spirits. It is important to remember that depression is a fairly common illness in the general population, particularly among the elderly.

In part, any depression can be overcome with a combination of cultivating positive attitude through support, counselling, and education about Parkinson's. In addition, some people with Parkinson's (just like many other people in the general population) may benefit from drug treatment for depression, and doctors may advise such treatment even for people who would not think of themselves as being depressed (we have discussed in the previous two questions how difficult it can be for any of us to recognize that we are either stressed or depressed).

The drugs commonly used to treat depression, known as antidepressants, are often used to treat depression in Parkinson's. However, some types are contraindicated in people with Parkinson's. See the PDS information sheet *Depression* (FS56) for more information.

Does Parkinson's affect the memory?

Sometimes memory difficulties can occur with Parkinson's. However, Parkinson's is often first diagnosed in people who are over the age of 55 – an age when many people have noticed that in any case their memory is not as good as it was!

Fortunately, many compensate with the cunning of experience!

The other problem in answering this question is that once any of us start thinking about our memories, we can all find many things that we feel we ought to remember. The shock of developing any illness at all, particularly when it leads to some depression, would make anybody more introspective and so liable to make a mountain out of a molehill as far as memory is concerned. Memory problems can be a sign of depression and of anxiety.

Some of the rarer drugs given for Parkinson's, particularly *anticholinergics* such as benzhexol (previously known as Artane), can affect memory and for this reason they are not usually prescribed for elderly people (there is more information about anticholinergics in the section on **Other Parkinson's drugs** in Chapter 3). They are sometimes prescribed in younger people with Parkinson's, but this is not common practice as they can also cause memory problems in younger people as well.

There are, however, some people with Parkinson's in whom serious and obvious memory problems raise concerns about more general mental deterioration.

Is there a link between Parkinson's and Alzheimer's?

This is a straightforward question to which it is impossible to give a straightforward yes or no answer.

Alzheimer's is the commonest cause of *dementia* (sometimes called brain failure), in which the brain cells die more quickly than in normal ageing. The main symptoms are loss of memory and the loss of the ability to do quite simple everyday tasks. The cells affected in Alzheimer's are not the cells in the substantia nigra that are affected in Parkinson's.

As Parkinson's and Alzheimer's are both more common in elderly people, if you look at a group of elderly patients with Parkinson's, you will find a proportion who do have memory loss, confusion, and disorientation in time and space – a type of dementia. This would be a higher number than if you looked at another group of elderly people who did not have Parkinson's. There are probably several reasons for this, including the drugs used to treat Parkinson's. Nearly all the drugs used can cause confusion in some people, although the anticholinergic drugs are especially suspect (there is more information about anticholinergics in the section on *Other Parkinson's drugs* in Chapter 3). When Parkinson's drugs are to blame, people usually get visions or other sorts of hallucinations, and if these are distressing, it may be necessary to change or withdraw the medication.

Sometimes, Parkinson's does affect the thinking parts of the brain, and so leads to other kinds of dementia. One type, called cortical *Lewy body disease*, has become better understood in recent years, and may account for many of the people who have symptoms of both Parkinson's and dementia early in the course of the illness. People with this condition are particularly prone to get early side effects like hallucinations, so the dose of the drugs given may be more cautious. Some patients may respond to the acetylcholinesterase inhibiting drugs more commonly tried in Alzheimer's disease. These include donepezil (Aricept), galantamine (Reminyl), rivastigmine (Exelon), and memantine (Ebixa). The latter has a slightly different mechanism of action. These drugs are usually prescribed via a memory clinic and patients are assessed carefully as to whether they are suitable and whether they respond. The Alzheimer's Society and Alzheimer Scotland – Action on Dementia can provide more information on all kinds of dementia (see Appendix 1 for contact details). The PDS has an information sheet on *Dementia and Parkinson's* (FS58).

I suffer badly from hair loss and my skin is constantly greasy. Could this be connected with my Parkinson's?

We don't know if you are a man or a woman, but in either case hair loss is not a particular feature of Parkinson's. In a man hair loss may be a natural effect of ageing (please see one of the authors!). In a woman it might be related to a general health problem, and we would suggest that you have a word with your GP.

A greasy skin can happen with Parkinson's but is not common and advice about careful skin care may help. Try washing with a mild, unperfumed soap and, if excessive dandruff is also a problem, you could try one of the special preparations, such as Selsun, available from the chemist. If the greasiness leads to irritation, you could ask your doctor to consider prescribing one of the lotions for dermatitis.

Can Parkinson's affect my eyes? I have got new glasses but still seem to have difficulty focusing sometimes.

Parkinson's does not directly affect the eye itself or the circuits for vision in the brain. However, the movements of the eyes can be affected to a slight degree in Parkinson's. This can lead to some problems turning the eyes inwards, which is necessary for reading. Any problems with focusing can usually be overcome by new glasses prescribed by a good optician who knows that you have Parkinson's.

Some Parkinson's medication (usually the anticholinergics) can cause poor focusing, as can some antidepressants. If you have recently started on any of these drugs, it would be worth asking your GP whether they could have anything to do with your eye problems. As with many other problems, you should not automatically assume that your Parkinson's is the culprit.

If your visual problems are more serious than those we have discussed, and your optician or GP cannot explain them, you should ask to be referred to an eye specialist for an opinion. PDS has an information sheet on *Eyes and Parkinson's* (FS27).

I can cope with the Parkinson's but get a lot of discomfort from constipation which seems to have got worse since I was diagnosed. Could there be a connection?

Yes, there could be a connection. Constipation is a very common complaint among people with Parkinson's, although often (as in your case) there has been a tendency to it beforehand. We would have hoped that your treatment for Parkinson's might have improved things a little but that does not seem to be the case. It may be that you have been prescribed one of the Parkinson's drugs which can make constipation worse. These include the anticholinergics, so if you have been prescribed one of these it might be worth having a word with your doctor (there is more information about anticholinergics in the section on *Other Parkinson's drugs* in Chapter 3).

Eating a healthy diet is important for everyone with Parkinson's and can also help with constipation (see Chapter 10 on *Eating and diet*). Medication for your constipation is necessary and important if you are getting a lot of pain, and your doctor or your chemist can advise you about this. Try not to get too anxious about how often you open your bowels, though we do understand how this can happen when you have had painful bouts of constipation. See the PDS information sheet on *Constipation* (FS80) The PDS booklets on *Diet* (B65) and *Looking After Your Bladder and Bowel* (B60) also include information on constipation.

My husband suffers badly from cramp, especially at night. Could this be anything to do with his Parkinson's?

Ordinary muscle cramps can certainly be a painful problem. They may respond to treatments such as quinine (from your doctor), to vigorous massage or simply to moving around.

However, there is a second type of leg cramp in which the foot turns inwards and for which the above treatments are unlikely to be as effective. It is also fairly common, but usually happens in the morning rather than at night. It is this type of cramp, known as dystonia, which is found most frequently in Parkinson's (although both types occur). If your husband's cramp is dystonia, then you will probably find that his foot gets stuck in one position. See the PDS information sheet, *Muscle Cramps and Dystonia* (FS43).

So what is dystonia and is it related to Parkinson's?

Dystonia is an involuntary contraction of the muscles which causes the affected part of the body to go into a spasm. In Parkinson's, it is seen most frequently in the leg (when the foot turns inwards) and then, but much more rarely, in the eyes (which cannot be opened easily). Dystonia can also affect the neck (so that it twists) or the hand and fingers (when the wrist usually bends at an angle). These dystonias do not appear to be caused by drugs and are a feature of the illness. We know this because very occasionally they are seen even before Parkinson's treatment has started.

Treatment for dystonia is not always easy. However, as dystonia in Parkinson's can be a sign of not enough medication, if you have this problem, it would be worth talking to your doctor to see if you could try increasing your dose. See the PDS information sheet *Muscle Cramps and Dystonia* (FS43).

My mother who is 84 and has had Parkinson's for many years has begun to get very restless and has 'jumpy legs'. Is this likely to be part of the Parkinson's or is it something else?

Your mother's symptoms are likely to be part and parcel of her Parkinson's. Such movements are common in people who have had the condition for many years. Nobody fully understands them, but they are partly a side effect of the *dopamine replacement therapy* and partly the result of some progression of the condition. Early in the course of the illness, doctors try to prevent them by adjusting the medication but, later on, it may be impossible to avoid them without causing increased slowing or freezing.

These movements are known by a number of different names – *involuntary movements* is the most straightforward and the one we have used in this book, but you may also hear them referred to as *dyskinesias* or *choreiform movements*. They can affect most of the body or just one part of it, and may affect different parts at different times. They can appear at certain times of the day, and when they occur is sometimes (although not always) linked to the timing of the last dose of dopamine replacement medicine (i.e. Madopar or Sinemet). We discuss the link between involuntary movements and treatment further in Chapter 3.

There are two other unlikely – but possible – causes for the symptoms you describe. The first is that they are common in drug-induced Parkinson's (there is more information about this condition in Chapter 1). The second is that there is another medical condition called *restless leg syndrome*. Nobody understands what causes it and it also occurs in people who do not have Parkinson's, when it occasionally responds to a different type of medication called clonazepam, but also to levodopa and dopamine agonists. PDS has an information sheet called *Restless leg syndrome* (FS83).

My husband who has Parkinson's is 82 and has developed a new and distressing symptom. Every afternoon he starts getting very hot and feels an inner – not outer – burning. He becomes very distressed and his breathing is affected. It used to go on for a few hours and a rest in bed seemed to relieve him, but in the last few days he has taken longer to recover.

The symptoms your husband is getting are not well understood by doctors, but they are recognized as being a part of Parkinson's. They appear to be both part of the Parkinson's itself, and a reaction to the drugs used to treat Parkinson's. However, stopping the drugs altogether (even when it is possible) rarely helps. Sometimes, but not always, this symptom occurs when people are getting involuntary movements (dyskinesias).

We are sorry to have to say that there is very little that can be done to relieve this symptom. We can, however, reassure your husband that it is not a sign of his Parkinson's getting worse or of another illness. We hope that this reassurance is of some help and that it may relieve some of the understandable anxiety which you are both feeling.

My wife has had Parkinson's for 10 years and has recently lost a lot of weight. The doctor says that there is nothing else wrong but she cannot seem to put on any weight. Is this a common problem?

People with Parkinson's sometimes lose 10 or even 20 pounds in weight. Weight loss can occur at any stage and often happens over a fairly short period and then stabilizes. It appears to be part of the Parkinson's and is hardly ever a separate cause for concern. This is even more likely to be the case if your wife has not lost her appetite. If, however, she has gone off her food, then it could be that she is suffering from depression and that her doctor should consider treatment for this. It may also be worth checking that she hasn't got swallowing problems. See the next question.

You do not say if your wife is getting involuntary movements. These can be a cause of weight loss in Parkinson's, as all movement uses up the energy that we take in from our food. It does not matter if the movement is involuntary or if we choose to take exercise, it all has the same effect.

Overall, if your wife is eating a well balanced diet (see Chapter 10 on *Eating and diet* for more information about this), if her own doctor is satisfied that there is no other cause for concern, and if her weight loss does not go on and on, we feel that it is best for you just to accept your wife's new weight and not make a thing of it. Forcing her to eat more can become self-defeating. See the PDS booklet on *Diet* (B65).

I have had Parkinson's for nine years and just recently have had some problems with swallowing. It is very embarrassing and distressing. What could be causing it?

Swallowing problems are not that common in the early years, but if you have had Parkinson's for nine years, then Parkinson's is the likely culprit. Nevertheless, as it is not common, doctors normally advise an examination by a throat specialist to make sure there is no other cause. It could, for example, be an easily treatable condition such as a piece of food or other foreign body stuck in the throat. However, if the specialist does not find anything (and they usually do not), then advice from a speech and language therapist can be very helpful, as he or she can teach you some 'tricks' that may help.

Once you have had this happen a few times, you may get into a vicious cycle of getting overanxious about it. The therapist can help you feel more in control and so get back to eating more normally. You will find information about how to get in touch with a speech and language therapist in Chapter 4 on *Access to treatment and services* and some more information on dealing with your problem in the section on *Eating and swallowing* in Chapter 9.

Is it true that 'pure' Parkinson's is rare and that most people with Parkinson's also have other conditions as well?

Yes, this is an inevitable consequence of the fact that Parkinson's mainly affects people over 60. The older you are when you get Parkinson's, the more likely you are to already have other medical conditions as well. After your diagnosis, you will not be immune from getting other illnesses, so every symptom you have should not be blamed on your Parkinson's. It can be quite difficult to sort out the overlapping symptoms but anything new should be discussed with your doctor and properly investigated. Problems with eyesight, bladder, swallowing or confusion can all be caused by Parkinson's, but they can also be caused by other things for which there are specific, effective treatments.

3
Treatment

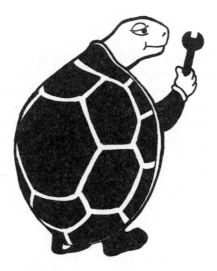

This chapter will deal with a variety of treatments, concentrating on the standard types (drug treatment and the *physical therapies*) but also touching on surgical interventions and on the wide range of complementary therapies.

Parkinson's is one of the few neurological conditions for which specific drug treatments are available and, although they do not cure the condition or halt its underlying progression, they can make a huge difference to the symptoms and greatly improve people's quality of life. It is important to remember the point we made in our introduction to this book (and have repeated several times since!) – that Parkinson's varies greatly from one person to another. It is impossible for anyone to suggest any one treatment which would be right for everyone. Two people whose symptoms look similar and who have been diagnosed for approximately the same length of time may need different drugs and different doses.

The same is true for the physical therapies. We can give an overview, but there will be individuals who are not helped by the therapies that help most people, and others who seem to respond to treatments which are generally considered to have little value. The important thing is to work together with your specialist, GP and other members of the health team to discover what works for you or your relative.

Levodopa, Sinemet and Madopar

What is the most frequently used drug treatment for Parkinson's?

The most frequently used drugs are co-careldopa (Sinemet) and co-beneldopa (Madopar). Both of these drugs contain *levodopa*, a compound one step removed from dopamine, the chemical messenger which is in short supply in Parkinson's (you will find more information about dopamine in Chapter 1). Once the levodopa reaches the brain it is changed into dopamine, so making up for the shortage. Sinemet and Madopar are therefore a form of replacement therapy – like insulin in the treatment of diabetes. The various versions of Sinemet and Madopar, together with some other rarely used forms of levodopa, are listed in Table 3.1 which gives both their trade and generic names, and the forms and sizes in which they are available.

Although these two drugs are the most used, not everyone with Parkinson's takes them. There are several other drugs available which may be more appropriate for some individuals at certain stages, and we discuss these later in this chapter.

Here are some comments on the drugs listed in the table:

- LS means low start: these versions of the drugs contain a small amount of levodopa and are often used in the early stages of treatment.

Table 3.1 Drugs containing L-dopa

Trade name	Generic name capsules	Tablets or capsules (mg)	Sizes available
Sinemet	co-careldopa	Tablets	110, 125, 275
Sinemet LS	co-careldopa LS	Tablets	62.5
Sinemet CR	co-careldopa CR	Tablets	250
Half Sinemet	co-careldopa CR	Tablets	125
Stalevo	levodopa/carbidopa/entacapone	Tablets	50
Stalevo	levodopa/carbidopa/entacapone	Tablets	100
Stalevo	levodopa/carbidopa/entacapone	Tablets	150
Madopar	co-beneldopa	Capsules	62.5, 125, 250
Madopar dispersible	co-beneldopa	Tablets	62.5, 125
Madopar CR	co-beneldopa CR	Capsules	125
Brocadopa	L-dopa	Capsules	125, 250, 500
Laradopa	L-dopa	Tablets	500

- CR means *controlled release,* and we discuss these versions of the drugs later in this section.

- Co-careldopa is a shorthand way of saying 'levodopa with carbidopa', and co-beneldopa 'levodopa with benserazide'.

- Carbidopa and benserazide are examples of *dopadecarboxylase inhibitors*, which are discussed later in this section.

- Stalevo is levodopa and carbidopa, i.e. Sinemet, combined with entacapone, the COMT inhibitor.

- Brocadopa and laradopa are hardly used nowadays, so do not be surprised if you have not heard of them before.

What is the difference between Sinemet and Madopar?

Both Sinemet and Madopar contain two separate kinds of drug. The first, as explained in the previous answer, is levodopa.

The second drug is there to prevent the side effects caused by taking levodopa on its own. To make use of the levodopa, the body has to change it into dopamine, and it can do this because it also makes another substance called dopa-decarboxylase. When levodopa was first discovered, it was given on its own but, because it was being changed in the bloodstream before reaching the brain, there were unpleasant side effects, particularly vomiting and low blood pressure. The discovery of other compounds which would stop the dopa-decarboxylase working until the blood carrying the levodopa reached the brain was an important breakthrough in preventing these side effects. For obvious reasons, these compounds are called dopa-decarboxylase inhibitors.

Sinemet and Madopar use different dopa-decarboxylase inhibitors: the inhibitor in Sinemet is called carbidopa, and the one in Madopar is called benserazide. However, the important thing to understand is that, as far as the brain is concerned, both drugs produce the same amount of dopamine. In spite of this, among the few people who have tried both Sinemet and Madopar, there are some who have a preference for one or the other. However, there is rarely any need to swap from one to the other.

What advantages do the 'controlled release' versions of Madopar and Sinemet offer?

We first ought to explain the difference between the 'ordinary' versions of these drugs and the controlled release versions. When you swallow the ordinary version of Sinemet or Madopar, the amount of the drug in your bloodstream rises in about half an hour, and then drops over the next hour or so. The controlled release versions simply keep the amount of the drug in your bloodstream at a steadier level.

The new versions were developed when it was noticed that, after a few years of satisfactory treatment, people were getting less reliable benefits from their medication. Efforts were made to develop forms of Sinemet and Madopar that remained at a more steady level in the bloodstream, and the result was the controlled release versions of these drugs. They do succeed in keeping the drug in the bloodstream for longer but the effect on fluctuating symptoms has been somewhat disappointing. Many people still need the 'kick start' of the ordinary forms where, although the drug goes up and down in the bloodstream faster, it goes up higher than with the controlled release drugs. Some people will, however, get a more even response to their doses of medication if they take the controlled release versions, although most will need to take a mixture of controlled release and ordinary Madopar or Sinemet.

Some people who notice troublesome symptoms at night will find that these controlled release drugs can be helpful, as they have a longer lasting effect. They are therefore most often used for the last dose of the day. Some specialists give them right from the beginning of treatment, when they work just as well as the ordinary versions.

Will I feel better straight away when I start taking Madopar?

The levodopa group of drugs such as Madopar or Sinemet often work fairly quickly. Many people, but by no means everyone, will feel some benefit within a few hours or days. However, even if you do not get an immediate effect, you are likely to notice some improvement over a week or two. If by chance you still don't feel much better then, you need to review the situation with your doctor. Sometimes your doctor will want to build up the dose slowly over several months.

What kinds of side effects do you get with Sinemet and Madopar?

Because these drugs put a natural compound back into the body, side effects at the beginning of treatment are rare. In the 1960s, when levodopa was given alone, vomiting and low blood pressure (with consequent fainting) were common. However, as explained earlier in this chapter, the addition of the dopa-decarboxylase inhibitors in Sinemet and Madopar has largely resolved these problems. Some people still get slight nausea or a little flushing right at the beginning of treatment.

A few people are very sensitive to the drugs and decide to discontinue them. However, if you are one of these people, do not exclude the possibility of trying an levodopa preparation a second time. Sometimes people in this situation do very well on their second attempt by starting with a lower than normal dose and building it up slowly.

Too much Sinemet or Madopar can cause involuntary movements (there is more information about involuntary movements in Chapter 2 and in the section on *Long-term problems* later in this chapter). Everything possible should be done to avoid this in the early years of treatment, but later on it may be necessary to put up with some involuntary movements in order to remain mobile. Such movements are not a simple side effect of the drugs but rather a mixture of the effects of the disease and of the medication. The same is true for the phenomena known as 'wearing off' and the 'on/off' syndrome (discussed in the section on *Long-term problems* later in this chapter).

How do I know if the side effects are normal or not?

When the doctor first prescribes your drugs, he or she will probably explain what effects you may experience as your body adjusts to the medication. You may also have access to a short and straightforward booklet called *The Drug Treatment of Parkinson's Disease* which is published by the PDS. If you are in any doubt about what may happen, have a word with your doctor or specialist. With this, as with any other questions for your doctor, it can be a good idea to make a list of the points that you wish to make, so that you don't forget to raise them at your next appointment.

All drugs can have some side effects and these have to be balanced against the advantages in each individual case. As explained in the answer to the previous question, it is unusual for Sinemet and Madopar to cause serious side effects. If you get involuntary movements, especially in the early stages of treatment, you should consult your doctor, as your dose of medication may need to be reduced.

Dopamine agonists

My doctor says there are some other drugs called dopamine agonists which can help. How do they work?

Dopamine agonists (sometimes called *dopa-agonists*) work in a different way from the replacement drugs like Sinemet and Madopar. They do not provide extra dopamine; instead they stimulate the parts of the brain where the dopamine works (*agonist* is a term used for drugs which have a positive stimulating effect on particular cells in the body).

Table 3.2 lists the dopamine agonists that are currently available in tablet or capsule form. Bromocriptine (Parlodel) has been around for many years; the others, all of which seem to work equally well, have been developed more recently. Cabergoline (Cabaser) does not need to be taken as often as the other tablets, so may be more convenient for some people. *Apomorphine* (discussed later in this section) is also a dopamine agonist but is currently only available as an injection.

What are the main advantages and disadvantages of dopamine agonists?

There are two main advantages. First, dopamine agonists rarely cause involuntary movements (there is more information about involuntary movements in Chapter 2 and in the section on *Long-term problems* later in this chapter) in people who have never been on any form of levodopa. Because of this advantage, some doctors are already preferring to prescribe an agonist to newly diagnosed people and then adding levodopa later if necessary. By

Table 3.2 Dopamine agonists available as tablets or capsules

Trade name	Generic name	Sizes available (mg)
Parlodel	bromocriptine	1.0, 2.5, 5.0, 10.0
Revanil	lysuride	0.2
Celance	pergolide	0.05, 0.25, 1.0
Requip	ropinirole	0.25, 1.0, 2.0, 5.0
Cabaser	cabergoline	1.0, 2.0, 4.0
Mirapexin	pramipexole (containing pramipexole substance)	0.125, 0.25, 1.0 0.088, 0.18, 0.7

doing this they hope to manage with lower doses of the levodopa drug and therefore to reduce the risk of later problems such as involuntary movements and fluctuating responses to medication.

Secondly, because these drugs remain in the bloodstream and in the brain for longer than Madopar and Sinemet, they can be tried for people who are having a fluctuating or unpredictable response to those medicines.

The disadvantages of the tablet/capsule forms of dopamine agonists are that:

- most people find them less effective in removing their symptoms than Madopar or Sinemet;

- they have to be introduced slowly;

- they may make the drug regimes of elderly patients with other illnesses too complicated;

- some side effects such as sleepiness and hallucinations may be slightly commoner;

- rare, but serious, side effects such as fibrosis (a thickening and scarring of connective tissue) occur with some of them.

Because of this complex mix of advantages and disadvantages, dopamine agonists are rarely used on their own in the long term.

Many people who try them will finish up on a combination of a dopamine agonist and a reduced dose of Madopar or Sinemet.

Are the newer dopamine agonists less likely to cause side effects?

We cannot give a direct answer to this question, because a trial that directly compares the main dopamine agonists has never been done. However, there is little evidence that any one dopamine agonist has any advantage over the others – they all appear to work equally well and to have much the same side effects with the exception of the ergot derivative drugs, e.g. pergolide/cabergoline/lisuride/bromocriptine that can rarely cause fibrosis in the abdomen or lung. If these drugs are to be used, blood tests and a chest X-ray are advised; sometimes lung function tests are recommended and advice on symptoms to look out for given.

What type of person can benefit from apomorphine?

The people who seem to benefit most are those who have bad 'off' periods but who are reasonably well when 'on'. It does not help everyone, but it is now often tried with people who have 'off' periods of half an hour or more and who have not improved after adjustments to their ordinary medication. As apomorphine (Apo-go) currently has to be given by injection, the person with Parkinson's and his or her *carer* have to be able to cope with this and to learn how to do it. This sometimes involves staying in hospital for a few days, although an increasing number of potential users are now being assessed and trained on a day care or domiciliary (home) care basis.

What are the main advantages of apomorphine?

Apomorphine is a dopamine agonist which is given by injection rather than as a tablet. The main advantage of apomorphine is that it can act as a 'rescue treatment' when tablets or capsules fail to take effect. For people who are assessed as suitable, it will work within 10–15 minutes – much more quickly than tablets or capsules. Because of this predictable response, it can sometimes help people with Parkinson's to go on working for longer than would otherwise be possible.

Does apomorphine have disadvantages too?

Yes. Its main disadvantage is that at the moment it can only be given by injection (other methods of delivery have been tried but have so far proved ineffective). This means that both the person with Parkinson's and their main carer need to be willing and able to give the injections. The technique and the confidence to use it can be taught (as we explain later in this section), but there are people who feel unable to face the prospect of having or giving regular injections. It is important to involve the main carer (who may be a partner or a close friend or relative) because there may be times when the person with Parkinson's is too rigid or immobile to give the injection.

Apomorphine also causes nausea and vomiting but this problem has been largely overcome by giving another drug called domperidone (Motilium) beforehand. Some people can even manage without the domperidone after a few months. Domperidone is a safe drug and, although it makes the drug regime a little more complicated, this is not really a disadvantage.

Another disadvantage is that the site of the injections can become rather sore and irritated, especially when a *syringe driver* is used. This problem can be reduced by diluting the apomorphine with an equal amount of saline (a sterile salt solution).

Is apomorphine addictive?

No.

I have been told that I may need to use a syringe driver for my apomorphine injections. What is a syringe driver?

A syringe driver (one type is shown in Figure 3.1) is a small, battery driven pump, which can deliver continuous medication through a needle inserted under the skin of your lower abdomen or outer, upper thigh. The medication is then absorbed into your bloodstream and goes from there to your brain. The dose can be adjusted to suit you, and the pump itself is carried in your pocket or in a small pouch round your waist. You need to change the needle and its position each day to reduce the risk of your skin getting sore. A small number of people use their syringe drivers continuously day and night. If this is essential, the needle site must be changed every 12 hours.

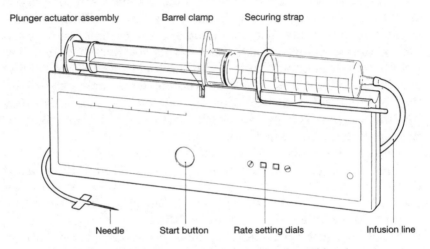

Plunger actuator assembly   Barrel clamp   Securing strap

Needle   Start button   Rate setting dials   Infusion line

Figure 3.1 One of the two main types of syringe driver in use

The proportion of people using a syringe driver rather than separate injections (see next question) varies with local and individual circumstances, but mainly they are people who need more than six injections a day. For them, the provision of a syringe driver can greatly improve the quality of life.

What are the alternatives to a syringe driver and how do they work?

There are two alternatives available at the moment. The first is a syringe of the type that people with diabetes use to give themselves their insulin. Some people who use apomorphine begin with this and many find it quite simple and easy to use. The syringe can be carried in a toothbrush container and fits easily into pockets and handbags.

The disadvantage of a syringe is that it can only hold one dose. For this and other reasons, some people prefer to use an injection pen, a special type of multidose syringe. Until recently the only pen available was the Hypoguard *Penject* which has to be loaded from the ampoules of apomorphine (Apo-go) prescribed by the pharmacist. This created a problem for some people, especially those living alone or with carers who were unable to carry out this task. Now Britannia Pharmaceuticals (see Appendix 1) has produced a ready-loaded, disposable Apo-go pen (see Figure 3.2), which overcomes this difficulty. It holds 30 mg of apomorphine and the individual dose (anything from 1 to 10 mg) is set by turning the dial. Britannia has issued clear and easy-to-follow booklets for patients and professionals.

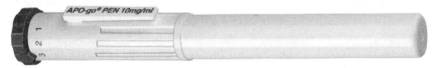

Figure 3.2 The ready-loaded, disposable Apo-go pen

The disadvantage of the Apo-go Pen is that it costs the Health Service considerably more than other methods, so clear evidence of the need for this particular method of injection should be provided by the consultant or Parkinson's Disease Nurse Specialist.

Both syringes and pens deposit the apomorphine (Apo-go) just under your skin, and have the advantage of not irritating it as much as a syringe driver. They do not, of course, give you continuous medication, but you can repeat your apomorphine injection several times a day as necessary.

How will I know which injection system is best for me?

Once the specialist has decided that you might benefit from apomorphine, the hospital team or Parkinson's Disease Nurse Specialist will decide which is the most appropriate system for you and will train you in its use. No one delivery system is right for everyone – the choice depends on many different factors like frequency of dose, manual dexterity, lifestyle and availability of help.

Can syringe drivers, syringes and injection pens be prescribed on the National Health Service?

There is little problem with prescribing the syringes as they are also widely used for diabetes. Apo-go pens can be prescribed but the needles come separately. These can be obtained free of charge by the pharmacist from Britannia Pharmaceuticals (who make apomorphine) as long as they are requested when you are ordering Apo-go pens.

Syringe drivers are available on loan from Britannia Pharmaceuticals free of charge. The syringes and fine infusion lines used with the syringe drivers are not obtainable on prescription. However, the syringes can be obtained free of charge from Britannia Pharmaceuticals as requested. The District Nursing Service pays for and provides the fine infusion lines. Your GP surgery can put you in touch with your local service.

Are there some special centres providing training and support to apomorphine users?

In several areas of the UK there are now *neurologists* or *geriatricians* (doctors who care for the elderly) with a particular interest in Parkinson's. In the hospitals or clinics where they work, there will generally be a special service for people who need apomorphine.

Many of these doctors work with Parkinson's Nurse Specialists (see Chapter 4 for more information on their role) and, if there is one, their role will include helping and supporting anyone who is trying apomorphine.

Are there any new developments in the pipeline which will make apomorphine easier to use?

Many people hope that a different method of delivering apomorphine (i.e. other than by injection) will be found. The most promising research is nasal delivery of apomorphine. *Clinical trials* of nasal sprays are currently taking place and there is a reasonable chance that they will become available in the foreseeable future. There are also other developments which could lead to delivery by mouth or via a skin patch. However, it is not clear yet whether such systems will offer the major advantage of injected apomorphine, which is its rapid action.

Other Parkinson's drugs

What other kinds of drugs are used in the treatment of Parkinson's?

So far we have discussed the drugs which contain levodopa and the dopamine agonists. There is another, older, group of drugs called anticholinergics which work by reducing the amount of another chemical messenger, *acetylcholine*, thereby slightly increasing the amount of dopamine activity. There are a large number of these anticholinergic drugs –the most commonly used are listed in Table 3.3.

Table 3.3 The most commonly used anticholinergic drugs

Trade name	Generic name
Akineton	biperiden
Broflex	benzhexol/trihexyphenidyl
Disipal	orphenadrine
Kemadrin	procyclidine

Although individuals may find one type or brand more suitable than another, in general no particular one stands out as better than the others. They are not used now nearly as much as they were before the discovery of levodopa, and they tend to be avoided for elderly people, as they can cause side effects such as confusion, dry mouth and difficulty in passing urine. Sometimes they are used alone in the early years before an levodopa preparation becomes necessary, but they are more frequently used as an addition to levodopa therapy. Anticholinergics can be useful to offset tremor or slowness of movement and can also be helpful when drooling (excessive salivation) is a problem.

It is not a good idea to stop anticholinergic drugs suddenly for any reason, including surgery, as this can lead to serious episodes of 'freezing' in which the person stops – as though rooted to the floor – and finds it difficult to get going again.

Amantadine (Symmetrel) is an old drug that has helped symptoms of Parkinson's disease a little. However, it has been shown that it is of benefit in some people in reducing involuntary movements and has recently been relaunched to help them.

What is the latest advice about selegiline? I keep hearing different things and am now completely confused. Is it a helpful drug or not?

It was originally thought that selegiline (Eldepryl/Zelapar) might have a two-fold beneficial effect. Firstly, by blocking the action of another chemical (*monoamine oxidase B*), which causes the breakdown of dopamine, it would allow more dopamine to be available to the brain. Secondly, in so doing, it would also reduce the amounts of potentially damaging compounds, known as *oxygen-free radicals*. As these compounds might be involved in killing off dopamine-producing cells, preventing the damage could perhaps slow down the natural progress of the disease. However, the current view is that this is not the case.

Anyone taking selegiline (Eldepryl/Zelapar) and later needing treatment for depression should ask their doctor to ensure that they are given an antidepressant suitable for use with MAOIs (the group of drugs to which selegiline belongs) as some should not be taken at the same time or within a few weeks of each other.

It is also important that anyone taking selegiline and needing to have a general anaesthetic should discuss any necessary temporary adjustments to their drug regime with their neurologist and surgeon. See PDS information sheet on *Anaesthesia* (FS36)

A new monoamine oxidase B inhibitor rasagiline is about to be marketed (Lundbeck with Teva Pharmaceuticals) with claims that it is more potent and less of a stimulant.

What are COMT inhibitors?

COMT (catechol-*O*-methyl transferase) inhibitors are a relatively new class of drugs for the treatment of Parkinson's. They work rather like selegiline (see answer to previous question) in that they block the action of a chemical which breaks down dopamine. Preventing this breakdown boosts the amount of dopamine available to the brain and also reduces the amount of the chemical by-product of the breakdown, which itself interferes with the action of dopamine. It is hoped that these new drugs (which are used with Sinemet or Madopar) will help people who are experiencing fluctuations in their response to medication, for example the wearing-off or the on/off phenomenon.

The first COMT tablet launched in Britain was tolcapone (Tasmar) in August 1997. Although not all those trying it benefited, some people reported very good results, so there was disappointment when, in November 1998, it was withdrawn from use throughout Europe. This action followed the deaths from hepatitis of three people taking the drug. (Hepatitis is a disease affecting the liver, and careful monitoring of liver function during the first six months of treatment had been an important aspect of the guidelines governing the use of this drug.) The drug is still available in USA and Switzerland and some people in the UK are prescribed it on a named patient basis.

Fortunately for those benefiting from the drug, another tablet in this same class of COMT inhibitors, entacapone (Comtess) was launched in Britain in September 1998, and has avoided similar problems, while being equally effective. Entacapone is given with each dose of Sinemet or Madopar. It is now being relaunched as a combined tablet with Sinemet, which will make it easier to take – its trade name is Stalevo. The indications for taking it will be the same and it will be given to people with fluctuations in their response to Sinemet alone in order to extend the action of the latter drug.

General questions about drug treatment

My friend, who has had Parkinson's for the same length of time as me, takes twice as many tablets as I do. Can this be right?

People with apparently similar types of Parkinson's can often need quite different doses. The dose required for any particular person has little to do with the severity of the symptoms or with the length of time since diagnosis. In other words, it is not good or bad to be on more or less drugs. The doses that are right for you and for your friend are the ones which give you the most benefit with the fewest side effects.

I was brought up to avoid taking tablets and often read of the damage they do. Now I have been diagnosed as having Parkinson's and have been told that I will have to take tablets for the rest of my life. Can I refuse?

You are, of course, free to decide not to take Parkinson's – or any other – drugs and you should always be involved in decisions about your health care. Before attempting a fuller answer to your question, we should acknowledge that there are quite a few people who feel as you do. Medicines are such a big part of health care today that it is easy for health workers to take them for granted and to underestimate the fears and feelings of people like yourself.

There are several important points to make. First you should explain to your doctor how you feel and ask him or her to set out for you the likely consequences of taking or not taking the medication. There is certainly no hurry to start medication in most people and there is still some controversy about the point at which drugs should be started and about which drugs should be used in early, mildly affected people. No doctor is therefore going to mind if you want to wait.

Secondly, it is worth remembering that drugs containing levodopa are a form of replacement therapy (putting back a natural compound) and they work reasonably well for most people. You might do yourself a disservice and reduce your quality of life if you wait too long.

Lastly, only you can know when the discomfort caused by your Parkinson's outweighs the discomfort you feel at being on permanent medication. Do not be afraid to return to your doctor if you decide to say no now but later want to change your mind.

Should I stop taking the tablets if they make me feel unwell?

We shall assume that you have been given an idea of what to expect in the early days of trying a new tablet. If you feel more unwell than you expected, for example if you feel very sick or faint, go back to your doctor as soon as possible and ask if you can stop taking those particular tablets. Your doctor may try you on a different sort of drug instead, or may suggest that you try the same drugs again but at a lower dosage. Some people do very well on their second attempt by starting with a lower than normal dose and building it up slowly.

Once you have settled on the tablets, particularly when they have proved helpful, it is usually unwise to change them suddenly. If you feel very unwell after a period of stable and successful treatment, the chances are that something other than the drugs is causing your new symptoms. Go to see your doctor so that you can explore what is causing the problem.

Can I adjust the tablets myself to suit my activities or how I am feeling?

When you have a good knowledge of your Parkinson's and know the difference between being underdosed and overdosed, many doctors will encourage you to experiment a little yourself with the precise dosage and timing of your tablets. Your doctor may, for example, be able to tell you that your total daily dose of Madopar or Sinemet should be roughly so many tablets and encourage you to experiment a little while keeping within this daily total. How you split them up during the day and how you take them in relationship to meals can be varied until, by a little trial and error, you find out what suits you best.

How important is the timing of medication in Parkinson's?

The timing is not too critical in the early years but, as time goes on, it becomes extremely important for many people with Parkinson's. This is because they can experience great discomfort and immobility (see the next section on *Long-term problems* for further discussion of these problems) and so need access to their medication at very precise times. This means that they have to plan their lives and activities very carefully – a loss of spontaneity which some people find very frustrating.

Problems with getting medication at the right times are especially acute when people with Parkinson's are admitted to hospital, especially when they are on non-neurological wards. The anxiety and distress caused by poor timing of their medication can add considerably to the normal stress experienced by people in hospital. Efforts are being made to increase understanding of these problems among medical and nursing staff – through seminars and through publications, such as the PDS information sheets on hospital admission for lay people and professionals, and their information pack for nurses – but we still hear accounts of bad experiences. We discuss ways in which people going into hospital can minimize these problems in Chapter 13.

I have heard that people should be started on dopamine agonists at first and not levodopa? Is this true? My mother who is 75 has been put on levodopa.

This is a controversial area. Several studies (including those called REAL-PET and CALM PD) were initially interpreted as showing that symptoms in people on dopamine agonists progressed slower than in those on levodopa. This argument is now disputed, although, as mentioned in answers to previous questions, some people on agonists do get fewer involuntary movements, often, however, at the expense of less benefit and increased chance of other side effects. It could be a case of six of one and half a dozen of the other, but at least the doctors have some choice and this should be discussed with you or your mother when treatment has already started. Despite heavy marketing of agonists, levodopa preparations still have a good case to be the initial treatment in some people: when symptoms are severe and a quick good response is necessary or, if drug regimens for other conditions are already complex enough, when the relatively simple dosage regimen of levodopa preparations is an advantage.

Studies, such as PDMED at the University of Birmingham, which randomize people between different classes of drugs are underway to try and answer these important questions. (See their website www.pdmed.bham.ac.uk for further information on PDMED).

I have read in the paper that drugs prescribed for Parkinson's can cause compulsive behaviour such as gambling. Is this true?

There have been reports in the newspapers following the publication of an article in *Neurology* (a scientific journal published by the American Academy of Neurology), which suggested that a rare side effect of dopamine agonist drugs, used to treat Parkinson's, may be compulsive gambling. There have also been a number of other small studies that have made a link between Parkinson's drugs and gambling.

Obsessive-compulsive behaviour has been observed in people with Parkinson's since before the advent of levodopa. Several structural and functional neuroimaging studies have shown that obsessive-compulsive disorder is related to dysfunction in the basal ganglia, the part of the brain affected in Parkinson's. Some researchers think that obsessive-compulsive behaviour may be an important but unrecognized feature in some people with Parkinson's and may be related to neurochemical changes in the basal ganglia in the brain that occur as Parkinson's progresses. A study conducted in Spain found a higher rate of obsessive-compulsive symptoms in people with advanced Parkinson's disease than those with early Parkinson's and other small studies have reported similar findings in the last three years.

Low levels of the neurotransmitter serotonin are believed to be involved in obsessions and compulsions. Drugs that increase the brain concentration of serotonin often improve obsessions and compulsions. Serotonin is also believed to play a role in Parkinson's and is the subject of ongoing research.

Excessive dopamine is also known to cause unusual behaviours. High doses of levodopa and dopamine agonists can occasionally cause behavioural problems, such as obsessive-compulsive behaviour and hypersexuality. However, it must be stressed that these side effects are very rare and, where they do occur, a reduction in dose or change of medication can resolve the problem.

Is it all right to take other kinds of medicines at the same time as those for Parkinson's?

People with Parkinson's often have other conditions for which they need medication. Reassuringly, the drugs for Parkinson's are not upset by other kinds of medication. It is particularly important to stress that, if people with Parkinson's become depressed, there is no reason for them to avoid normal antidepressant drugs if their doctors think that these will be helpful. You can also take painkillers and sleeping pills.

There are, however, a number of drugs (listed in Table 3.4) which should almost always be avoided by people with

Table 3.4 Drugs to be avoided or questioned if they are prescribed

Trade name	Generic name	Prescribed for
Stemetil	prochlorperazine	Dizziness
Maxolon	metoclopramide	Vomiting
Fluanxol	flupenthixol	Depression
Motipress Motival	fluphenazine and nortriptyline	Depression
Parstelin	tranylcypromine and trifluoperazine	Depression
Triptafen	amitriptyline and perphenazine	Depression
Anquil	benperidol	Hallucinations/Mild confusion or disorientation/ Disturbed thinking
Clopixol	zuclopenthixol	Hallucinations/Mild confusion or disorientation/ Disturbed thinking
Depixol	flupenthixol	Hallucinations/Mild confusion or disorientation/ Disturbed thinking
Dolmatil	sulpiride	Hallucinations/Mild confusion or disorientation/ Disturbed thinking
Dozic	haloperidol	Hallucinations/Mild confusion or disorientation/ Disturbed thinking
Droleptan	droperidol	Hallucinations/Mild confusion or disorientation/ Disturbed thinking
Fentazin	perphenazine	Hallucinations/Mild confusion or disorientation/ Disturbed thinking
Haldol	haloperidol	Hallucinations/Mild confusion or disorientation/ Disturbed thinking

Table 3.4 Drugs to be avoided or questioned (*continued*)

Trade name	Generic name	Prescribed for
Largactil	chlorpromazine	Hallucinations/Mild confusion or disorientation/ Disturbed thinking
Loxapac	loxapine	Hallucinations/Mild confusion or disorientation/ Disturbed thinking
Melleril	thioridazine	Hallucinations/Mild confusion or disorientation/ Disturbed thinking
Moditen	fluphenazine	Hallucinations/Mild confusion or disorientation/ Disturbed thinking
Neulactil	pericyazine	Hallucinations/Mild confusion or disorientation/ Disturbed thinking
Orap	pimozide	Hallucinations/Mild confusion or disorientation/ Disturbed thinking
Serdolect	sertidole	Hallucinations/Mild confusion or disorientation/ Disturbed thinking
Serenace	haloperidol	Hallucinations/Mild confusion or disorientation/ Disturbed thinking
Sparine	promazine	Hallucinations/Mild confusion or disorientation/ Disturbed thinking
Stelazine	trifluoperazine	Hallucinations/Mild confusion or disorientation/ Disturbed thinking
Sulparex	sulpiride	Hallucinations/Mild confusion or disorientation/ Disturbed thinking
Sulpitil	sulpiride	Hallucinations/Mild confusion or disorientation/ Disturbed thinking

Parkinson's. This is because they tend to bring on Parkinson's-like symptoms. The list includes some of the antidepressant drugs, but there are many alternative ones available.

A word of caution is necessary here. We cannot guarantee that the list of drugs given in Table 3.4 is exhaustive, as new drugs are being developed all the time. If you are offered a new drug by your doctor (or any drug which you have not had before, for that matter), it is always worth asking whether it is suitable for someone with Parkinson's.

Some of the newer antipsychotics are believed to have fewer side effects acting on the part of the brain affected by Parkinson's, which is why they will be given with caution in people with Parkinson's who hallucinate. However, these drugs can still make the Parkinson's worse, so they will be prescribed very carefully and usually at a low dosage. Recent research has suggested that two of the newer antipsychotic drugs, risperidone (Risperdal) and olanzapine (Zyprexa), should be used with caution to treat dementia in people at risk of stroke (the risk increases with age, hypertension, diabetes, atrial fibrillation, smoking and high cholesterol levels) because of an increased risk of stroke and other cerebrovascular problems.

My brother has glaucoma. Does that mean that some Parkinson's drugs will not be available to him?

There is no major problem for people with glaucoma, especially if the glaucoma itself is being adequately treated. Anticholinergic drugs such as benzhexol (previously known as Artane) will probably have to be avoided, but these Parkinson's drugs are not used very much now anyway. There is no major problem with levodopa replacement therapy (Madopar and Sinemet) or with dopamine agonists (all discussed earlier in this chapter). The drugs your brother needs for his glaucoma will not upset his Parkinson's. It would helpful if the Parkinson's specialist and the ophthalmologist work together when prescribing medication for people like your brother who have Parkinson's and glaucoma. Anybody with glaucoma should always bring this fact to the attention of any doctor they see.

There is a PDS information sheet on *Eyes and Parkinson's* (FS27).

Does having a pacemaker create any problems in Parkinson's medication?

There should be no problem with a pacemaker. In the days before levodopa (i.e. treatment before we had Sinemet and Madopar), preparations included a dopa-decarboxylase inhibitor there were some potential problems, but not now. There is no problem with dopamine agonists either. When treatment for depression is also required, the *cardiologist* may be wary of some antidepressant drugs, depending on the particular cardiac condition you have.

Actually fitting and managing the pacemaker should cause no problems and cardiologists are well used to looking after people with other illnesses in addition to their heart complaints.

I have heard of people with Parkinson's having too much saliva, but I have a dry mouth which I find very uncomfortable. Why should this be?

Yes, people with Parkinson's sometimes have too much saliva, not because more than normal is being produced, but because the continual swallowing which we all do is slowed down, so the saliva accumulates in the mouth and can overflow. The dry mouth which you have is, however, likely to be related to your medication. This could either be an anticholinergic such as benzhexol or one of the antidepressants. Changing the dosage may be helpful but you have, of course, been given these drugs for a good reason, so you need to discuss the various options with your doctor. Once again it is a question of trying to find a fairly happy medium.

Sucking glycerine and honey sweets may help to make your mouth feel less dry, and ice cold water or citrus-flavoured drinks with or between meals can also be helpful.

Long-term problems

Why do some people with Parkinson's suffer from excessive movements of the head and body?

These are involuntary movements (as we mentioned in Chapter 2, they are also known as dyskinesias or choreiform movements). They vary greatly in their severity but are quite common, particularly in people who have had Parkinson's and been treated for it over a number of years. They are not well understood but seem to be part and parcel of an artificial increase in the dopamine in the brain. We know that they are not just a side effect of the drugs because, if people who do not have Parkinson's take these same drugs, they do not get these movements. They are partly caused by the Parkinson's and partly by the fluctuating levels of Madopar or Sinemet (there is a section about these drugs at the beginning of this chapter).

When involuntary movements appear, they are usually a sign that the dose of Madopar or Sinemet is on the high side, so a reduction in the dose is usually tried. However, this sometimes leads to a return of the Parkinson's symptoms of slowness and stiffness, and a new compromise between mobility and involuntary movements has to be sought.

The frequency and timing of the involuntary movements differs between individuals. In some, the movements are there most of the time, while in others they tend to appear just after taking a tablet or shortly before the next one is due. Some people find them very troublesome but, when they are fairly mild, they are often more upsetting to an observer than to the person with Parkinson's – as we discuss in the answer to the next question. The PDS has an information sheet on *Motor Fluctuations* (FS73).

My son's involuntary movements distress me greatly and I think he should take fewer tablets but he disagrees. What do you think?

Other people often notice involuntary movements more – and are more disturbed by them – than the person with Parkinson's. Your son's argument will be that if he reduces the dose he will feel underdosed and his Parkinson's symptoms will return. In such a situation, particularly if his movements were severe, we would encourage him to try a reduction in the dose. If he tries and he does feel and look worse, you may have to accept that he is better off with the involuntary movements than without them.

Your son does need to understand that his involuntary movements are a sign that he is on the top dose of treatment that he can take (or even that he is already just over the top), so he should not just take more and more tablets thinking that they will help. The misconception that more is better can lead, in some people, to an obsession with their medication and when the next dose is due. Although this is understandable when people are experiencing severe fluctuations, it can sometimes lead to them taking more drugs that is sensible. People who feel that their total daily dose of treatment is inadequate should discuss this with their doctor, and not simply increase the dose themselves.

My tablets do not seem to last as long as they used to so I have times, just before a dose, when I feel very slow and rigid. Why has this started to happen and what can be done to help?

What you are experiencing is fairly common after several years on levodopa replacement therapy (which is discussed in the first section of this chapter). It is known as the *'wearing off' phenomenon* for the obvious reason that the effectiveness of the medication 'wears off' before the next dose is due. There are various theories about why it happens but no satisfactory explanation exists at the moment. With drugs taken by mouth, the amount of the drug in the bloodstream goes up and down fairly quickly but, in the earlier years of Parkinson's, the brain is able to handle these fluctuations and give a fairly smooth response. However, as the years go by, the brain seems less able to do this and the benefit you get from your tablets starts to vary roughly in time with the level in the bloodstream.

There are several possible ways of trying to improve the situation, and you should talk to your doctor or specialist to see which one he or she recommends. There are four main options.

- Keep your total daily dose of Sinemet or Madopar about the same but take smaller doses more frequently.

- Take your tablets before, rather than with, meals so that the levodopa has less competition from the protein in your food, and/or try redistributing your daily protein (e.g. meat, cheese, eggs) so that most of it is taken at your evening meal rather than at mid-day, thus minimizing any disruption of your daytime activities. (Chapter 9 on *Eating and diet* includes more information about protein in your diet.)

- Consider changing to one of the controlled release forms of Madopar or Sinemet. They keep the levels in the bloodstream more constant and can reduce the fluctuations, but most people find that they need a mixture of the controlled release and ordinary forms of the drug.

- Consider adding entacapone (Comtess). This may help to keep the levels of drugs in the bloodstream more constant, although a reduction in the dose of Sinemet or Madopar may be necessary in some people to avoid increased involuntary movements. Alternatively, your doctor may switch you to the combined pill that contains entacapone, Stalevo.

If none of these works for you, your specialist might consider trying dopamine agonist tablets or capsules (there are questions about these drugs earlier in this chapter). If this is the chosen option, it may be necessary to reduce your dose of the levodopa preparation – otherwise you may start getting too many involuntary movements.

My wife has had Parkinson's for many years and now she can change from reasonable mobility to absolute immobility in minutes. What causes this sudden change?

Your question contains a very good description of something we call the *on/off phenomenon*. Some people call it *yo-yoing*. It usually happens with people (like your wife) who have had Parkinson's for five to 10 years or so. It is just as you describe, in that people can go from being quite well, with or without some involuntary movements, to becoming immobile, perhaps with recurrence of tremor, all in the space of a few minutes. This phase can last for quite some time and differs from the freezing (described in Chapter 2) which happens whilst walking and which lasts for seconds rather than minutes or hours.

The explanation of these fluctuations is, like the 'wearing off' phenomenon, not understood and is a major target for research. The current explanation is similar to that for the 'wearing off' phenomenon. In other words, as the years go, by people become very sensitive to the amount of the drug in their bloodstream and this triggers (sometimes very quickly) changes in symptoms from being 'on' (well and able to move around, with or without involuntary movements) to being 'off' (immobile with or without tremor).

Improving the situation is even more difficult than for the 'wearing off' phenomenon, although the same changes to treatment are usually tried (we have listed these in the answer to the previous question). Your wife's specialist may suggest that she tries an injected form of dopamine agonist called apomorphine (Apo-go) rather than a tablet form. There is more about apomorphine in the section on **Dopamine agonists** earlier in this chapter. The PDS has an information sheet on *Motor Fluctuations* (FS73) which includes information on on-off phenomenon and wearing off.

My mother has great difficulty in swallowing and getting her tablets down is becoming a major problem. Can anything be done to help?

Swallowing can be a problem with Parkinson's, although it is not very common in the early years. The doctor should check for other possible causes and might refer your mother to a throat specialist for advice. If your mother's problems turn out to be due to her Parkinson's, her medication could be reviewed. Anticholinergic drugs tend to cause a dry mouth which can exacerbate swallowing difficulties so, if she is taking any of these, her doctor might suggest gradually trying without them.

There are two other things that can be done. First of all, if she finds liquids easier to swallow than solids, there is a soluble form of Madopar called Madopar dispersible which can be dissolved in water. Some changes of dosage and timing may be necessary, and this will be explained by her doctor. There is no dispersible form of Sinemet: standard Sinemet tablets can be crushed prior to use and mixed with liquid or a spoonful of yoghurt, for example. This may make swallowing the tablets easier and speed the rate of their absorption. (Note that Madopar capsules should **not** be broken). There may be a short period of trial and error until she gets the same effect as with her previous tablets.

Her specialist or GP should also involve a speech and language therapist in treating this problem. They have a special interest in swallowing and can often suggest ways of easing the problem.

There is some more information about swallowing problems in Chapter 10 on *Eating and diet* and there is also a PDS information sheet (*Drooling and swallowing*, FS22).

My elderly mother is constantly drooling. What can be done to help?

Overflowing saliva (*drooling* or *dribbling*) is quite common in advanced Parkinson's. It happens, not because too much saliva is produced, but because Parkinson's slows the natural tendency to swallow and also makes poor lip closure and a bent posture more likely.

There are no easy solutions. The anticholinergic drugs (discussed earlier) and some of the drugs used for depression can help, but anticholinergic drugs can have quite a lot of unwanted side effects, especially in elderly people. The same drugs – and also scopolamine (Scopoderm), used for travel sickness – can be given by skin patches but tend to have the same side effects as the tablets and may also cause sore skin.

Very occasionally surgery or radiation therapy on the salivary glands has been attempted. Although this treatment has been known for many years, it is rarely used as the results are unpredictable and can cause side effects, including an overdry mouth. Botulinum toxin injections are also being used by some doctors. See also the PDS information sheet *Drooling and swallowing* (FS22).

My husband who is in his seventies has been taking antiparkinson's drugs for many years. Lately, he has developed terrible nightmares and has hallucinations during the day – sometimes he maintains he can see soldiers marching through the room and so forth. Both of us find this very distressing. Can you explain what could be causing this and whether anything can be done to help?

Thank you for bringing up this problem which is not too uncommon, especially in people over the age of 70 who have had Parkinson's for a long time (as in your husband's case). As with many things that happen with Parkinson's, there is no simple explanation. We know that they are not just a side effect of the drugs because, if people who do not have Parkinson's take these same drugs, they do not get hallucinations. They are probably partly caused by the Parkinson's and partly by the drugs.

Virtually any of the drugs used to treat Parkinson's can be partly to blame. If your husband is on anticholinergics, most doctors would start by trying to reduce them, and then slowly stop them altogether. However, usually it is levodopa replacement therapy or a dopamine agonist which is to blame. In some people reducing these drugs can get rid of the problem, but this may result in increasing immobility. In this case a not very happy intermediate course has to be tried, aiming for reasonable mobility and some reduction in the hallucinations, but perhaps not eliminating them altogether. Although it sounds unlikely in your husband's case, some people do not find their hallucinations or dreams particularly upsetting so, for them, these difficult compromises are not necessary. If, on the other hand, distressing hallucinations and confusion continue even after significant reductions in the drugs, it could, sadly, mean the onset of dementia.

Drugs that are given to treat hallucinations in other diseases unfortunately tend to aggravate Parkinson's symptoms so may not help your husband. However, research is continuing into new drugs, which could overcome this problem. They include clozapine (Clozaril), and quetiapine (Seroquel, the current favourite), although all have other side effects and require careful monitoring. Some antipsychotic drugs seem to increase the risk of stroke in patients with dementia or other risk factors for stroke, and in particular, the advice is that risperidone and olanzapine are avoided. See also the PDS information sheet on *Hallucinations* (FS11).

Whatever the outcome of adjustments to your husband's drug regime, if you are not already receiving support and advice from your local health professionals, social services or from the Parkinson's Disease Society, we would strongly recommend that you seek out such help. You may also find some of the suggestions in Chapter 6, *Caring for the 'carers'*, helpful.

Physical therapies

I recently had a course of physiotherapy after a fall due to my Parkinson's and found it a great help. No one ever suggested it before. Why is it not more widely available?

Physiotherapy is of use with Parkinson's although clearly it cannot correct the whole problem. Many people have had a similar experience to yours – they have found physiotherapy extremely helpful after a fall or when they have been made immobile, perhaps because of an operation. In these situations, physiotherapy helps people to get going again and restores any confidence which they may have lost. It is also quite helpful in people who are having difficulty with their walking.

Physiotherapy is not often suggested in the very early stages of Parkinson's, although there are some people (including one of the authors and several physiotherapists!) who think that an early referral for assessment and advice on exercises and self-help can have important, long-term advantages. Usually people are just advised by their doctors to keep as active as possible.

In general we agree that referrals for physiotherapy are not made as often as they should be, partly because there is a shortage of physiotherapists but also because there is lack of awareness about how helpful their intervention can be. Sometimes it is necessary to be very persistent and nag your GP or specialist even to get a trial course to see whether it helps or not. Access to physiotherapy is discussed in Chapter 4, and there are more examples of the use of physiotherapy in Chapter 9.

One of the most frustrating aspects of my Parkinson's is the way it interferes with so many everyday tasks from doing up buttons to getting out of chairs and turning over in bed. What help can I get with these problems?

Certainly the problems which you describe are amongst the most frustrating and difficult aspects of Parkinson's. Although the medication usually helps considerably, it does not always provide the complete solution, and then help from both physiotherapists and occupational therapists can be very useful. Sometimes it is a case of finding a new way of tackling problems and sometimes a question of identifying the right type of equipment. You will find many examples of the ways these therapists can help in Chapter 9, and information about getting access to them in Chapter 4.

Can speech therapy help people with Parkinson's?

Speech therapy (now called speech and language therapy) can be of benefit to some people with Parkinson's who are having problems with their speech, their facial expression or their swallowing.

There can be a range of speech problems, from low volume and hoarseness to difficulty in getting started or speaking too quickly, and it is important to get the help of a speech and language therapist with an interest in Parkinson's. As with other therapists, speech and language therapists sometimes feel that they are brought in too late to have maximum effect. Even in the early stages they can suggest exercises which improve facial mobility and expressive speech, and so help people retain good communication skills for longer than would otherwise be the case. There is more information on the ways in which they can help in Chapter 7 on *Communication*.

As we mentioned earlier in this chapter, speech and language therapists also have a special interest in swallowing and should be involved when this is causing problems. There is some more information about swallowing problems in Chapter 10 on *Eating and diet*.

The PDS has information on all the therapies described in the last three questions.

How might a dietitian be involved in the treatment of Parkinson's?

There are several possibilities here. When people are having the severe involuntary movements or 'on/off' symptoms we discussed earlier in this chapter, one approach that can be taken is to reduce or rearrange the protein in their food. Such dietary changes are best undertaken with the advice of a *dietitian*. Secondly, people with Parkinson's can be overweight or underweight, and in both cases the advice of a dietitian may be sought. Finally, when there are swallowing problems, the dietitian can suggest ways of preparing and presenting food and drink so that it is both nutritious and easier to swallow. (See Chapter 10 for more details on these matters.)

Surgical treatments

I have read that there used to be a surgical operation to reduce severe tremor. Is this ever carried out now, and if not, why not?

The operation which you read about is known as *stereotactic thalamotomy*. It involves putting a very fine needle into the brain and causing careful and selective damage to certain cells in the thalamus. The thalamus is a part of the brain (located near the substantia nigra) which is responsible for relaying information from the sense organs about what is going on in the body to the various parts of the brain. The objective of the operation is to improve the tremor by 'circuit breaking' some overactive circuits within this part of the brain.

These operations were done quite often before drug treatment with levodopa replacement therapy (Madopar and Sinemet) came along. They are done less often now, especially as brain surgery always carries some risk. In any event, the drugs are thought to work better than the operations, although they are perhaps less effective against tremor than against slowness and rigidity. The operation was better, as you say, at reducing tremor which, although less disabling than slowness and rigidity, can be extremely embarrassing. It can only safely be done on one side as speech often deteriorates when it is done on both sides.

The operation is still considered when tremor on one side of the body is the chief problem and the tremor has not responded to medication. As few people fall into this category, the operation has become a rarity.

There seems to be renewed interest in other operations called pallidotomy and subthalamotomy. Can you explain what these involve? Are they likely to be helpful to some people with Parkinson's?

Pallidotomy is another form of stereotactic surgery (see the *Glossary* for a definition of this term) which uses similar techniques to those described in the answer to the previous question to damage and so 'circuit break' some overactive circuits in a small area in another part of the brain called the pallidum. First carried out in the 1950s, it was rediscovered in the 1980s, and results suggest that it may be especially helpful to people who are getting severe involuntary movements, although it can also alleviate the symptoms of slowness, rigidity and tremor. Considerable numbers of people with severe involuntary movements (dyskinesia) are now having a pallidotomy on one side of the brain although, because there is a risk of stroke, the decision is never an easy one. Operations on both sides can be performed, but carry an increased risk of slurred speech and swallowing difficulties. They are therefore best avoided if these problems are already present.

Subthalamotomy is a newer but similar operation, which targets a different and smaller part of the brain called the *subthalamus*. Results look less promising than originally thought, and it is not currently being performed in the UK, although it may be offered in countries that do not have the expertise or resources for deep brain stimulation (see below).

I have heard of pacemakers for the brain. Do these work in Parkinson's?

Yes, the use of pacemakers in the treatment of Parkinson's was pioneered in France and has now spread to other countries, including the UK. The proper name for this type of surgery is *deep brain stimulation*. A wire, connected to an implantable pulse generator (IPG) is implanted in the chosen area of the brain (initially the pallidum, but now increasingly the subthalamus), The IPG is then implanted under the skin in the chest. It produces the electrical signals for the stimulation and can be turned on and off by the person with Parkinson's using a small magnet.

Deep brain stimulation is costly, and only a proportion of people with Parkinson's are suitable for the treatment, but the results look impressive. It is like pallidotomy and subthalamotomy (discussed in the previous question) in that it is helpful to people with disabling involuntary movements, whilst also alleviating the basic Parkinson's symptoms. These pacemakers may provide an advance in treatment over the next few years, but they need a large investment of patient and staff time to make them work well. Trials using quality of life and economic measures are under way in five centres in the UK and another five will join in shortly. People are included in these trials who:

- have good general health with no signs of dementia;

- have usually had Parkinson's for 6–12 years;

- responded well initially to drugs but are now fluctuating with quite severe dyskinesia at times;

- have 'off' periods but at some point of the day are well controlled.

The response to the stimulation of the brain cells is enough for the doctor to usually be able to reduce the drug dosage, which is why the involuntary movements are lessened.

I would like to know more about fetal cell transplantation surgery – can you give me some information?

Yes – we discuss it in Chapter 14 on *Research and clinical trials*, along with other surgical techniques that are being researched.

The PDS has a booklet on *Surgery and Parkinson's* (B78).

Complementary therapies

Do doctors disapprove of complementary or alternative medicines?

Before trying to answer this question, we need to make a distinction between medicines or therapies which claim to be 'alternatives' to the treatment offered by the medical profession, and those which are 'complementary' and are meant to be used alongside conventional treatments. The use of a *complementary therapy* should be in addition to, and not instead of, your usual treatment – no one should stop taking their normal drugs without a doctor's approval.

Doctors in general are happier with the idea of complementary therapies. The medical profession seems to be becoming more sympathetic to these therapies, some of which are very ancient, and is perhaps also more aware of the shortcomings in what it has to offer in some situations. At the same time, the reputable members of these various therapies are trying harder to improve their own practices and to give the public more information about their qualifications and training. The Complementary Medical Association and the Institute for Complementary Medicine (see Appendix 1 for addresses) are useful sources of further information, or you can enquire at your own GP surgery or health centre for the names of reputable local practitioners. Some GP practices now offer certain complementary therapies themselves.

The reservations held by many members of the medical and health professions largely revolve around the fact that very few of these treatments have been subjected to properly controlled trials. This means that there is little hard evidence that the treatments really work. Various efforts are being made to address this problem. There is now a Research Council for Complementary Medicine, and the University of Exeter has the first Professor of Complementary Medicine in Europe. The PDS Complementary Therapy Working Group has produced detailed guidelines to help researchers – these are available from the PDS.

Doctors get upset about alternative or complementary medicines when people are tempted to stop their normal treatment, when the therapies have serious side effects, and when they feel that their patients are being misinformed and persuaded to spend large sums of money which they can ill afford. If these features are not present, most practising doctors will take a benign view of these forms of therapy and appreciate that, even if the scientific evidence or rationale for them is elusive, they may well do some good. This is especially likely if the people concerned feel enthusiastic about them. They may

give people a sense of doing something for themselves which can
be very valuable and may also help them to relax.

The following questions and answers cover the main
complementary therapies that either have been researched in
relation to Parkinson's or people with Parkinson's regularly ask
for information about. The PDS has a booklet on *Complementary
Therapies* (B73), from which much of the information in this
section is taken.

I like the idea of music therapy. What does it have to offer people with Parkinson's?

Music therapy sounds delightful and certainly has no harmful side
effects. Many people with Parkinson's discover for themselves
that listening to strong rhythmic music can improve their walking,
prevent hesitations, and overcome freezing episodes. Metronomes
have also been tried with some success. Some people find that
they are still able to dance even though walking is difficult and
that they tire less easily when moving to music.

Music with a regular beat and perhaps a tune which is familiar
or has some emotional significance seems to be the most helpful.
The skilled music therapist can use music in a structured way to
build on these observations. In this way, music therapy can help
with physical activities like walking and upper limb movements,
with involuntary movements and tremor, and with speech
disturbances. It can also reduce fatigue. Music therapists often
work on these problems with other therapists such as physiotherapists and speech and language therapists.

It is not necessary to have any musical experience to enjoy the
benefits of music therapy. The benefits are most obvious during
the therapy sessions, but preliminary studies suggest that there is
a significant 'carry-over' effect.

Unfortunately music therapists are rather thinly spread across
the UK and gaining access to them may be difficult. If you are
interested, contact the Association of Professional Music
Therapists (see Appendix 1 for the address) to see if there is one
working in your part of the country.

I love painting and drawing. Would art therapy help my Parkinson's?

Many people with Parkinson's love painting, drawing and other kinds of art and crafts activities, even if their symptoms sometimes make these activities difficult. We would encourage you to continue to enjoy painting and drawing. If you have specific difficulties, such as holding a paintbrush, an occupational therapist may be able to provide advice or suggestions on making things easier for you.

Art therapy helps to reduce stress by working on the subconscious. Techniques often focus on activities that stimulate the imagination, release frustration and encourage a meditative frame of mind. This might include doodling, drawing and painting to music, finger painting, and memory painting.

Research carried out in this area with people with Parkinson's has proved that many feel the benefit of art therapy.

The British Association of Art Therapists has a directory of qualified therapists working in the UK (see Appendix 2 for details).

Is hypnosis useful in overcoming Parkinson's symptoms such as tremor, 'off' periods and freezing?

We have probably all heard about the use of hypnosis in helping people break bad habits, such as smoking, and it is also sometimes used in illnesses which are thought to have a large psychological component (hypnosis is said to put you more in touch with your subconscious self). It may also help in conditions like Parkinson's which are aggravated by stress.

When you are hypnotized, you enter a state of very deep relaxation. People can be taught self-hypnosis, and some therapists may provide audiocassettes that you can listen to at home to help with this. In Parkinson's, it is most likely to help with stress management and in doing so help to reduce tremor, excessive sweating and, perhaps, involuntary movements. If it helps you to relax and cope with stress more effectively, it may also reduce the discomfort of 'off' periods and episodes of freezing.

If you feel that hypnosis might help you, discuss it with your GP who may be able to suggest a reputable practitioner. If this is not possible, follow the suggestions given in the first question in this section and consult one of the main complementary medicine organizations for advice.

Is there any evidence that homeopathy can help in Parkinson's?

To our knowledge, there is no good evidence that *homeopathy* can help in any very specific way. However, as with the other complementary therapies, it tries to look at the person as a whole and, in so doing, may lead to overall improvements in well-being.

Some people say that osteopathy can help with Parkinson's symptoms. Is this true?

We can't give a definite answer to this question, partly because there are no carefully controlled studies of its use in Parkinson's but also because many people with Parkinson's have other conditions which may respond to osteopathy. Certainly there are osteopaths who feel that they have a contribution to make and people with Parkinson's who feel they have been helped. Many doctors accept that *osteopathy* can be helpful for the aches and pains to which people with Parkinson's are prone.

It is important to find a registered osteopath (see Appendix 1 for address of the General Osteopathic Council). Osteopathy is the first complementary therapy to become a regulated profession (in the same way that doctors, nurses and dentists are regulated). Since May 2000, it has been illegal for any therapist to claim that they are an osteopath unless registered with the General Osteopathic Council.

Would aromatherapy help my husband as he is in great discomfort in bed?

It is impossible to predict whether or not *aromatherapy* will help your husband. When aromatherapy is carried out properly, the major benefits seem to be physical and mental relaxation. This offers a number of potential benefits to those with Parkinson's, particularly for symptoms made worse by stress and for helping ensure a good night's sleep. If your husband's discomfort is due to inability to relax or to painful muscles and joints, it could be worth a try. There are two principal ways of using aromatherapy – smelling the oils using burners or adding a few drops to a bath, or through massage with *essential oils*. It is important to consult a properly qualified aromatherapist before you try aromatherapy to ensure that you are using them safely and effectively. Some essential oils are contraindicated for certain conditions and some commercially obtainable oils can be toxic for some people. The Aromatherapy Organizations' Council has a national register of aromatherapists for referral to the public.

More conventional approaches that might also help your husband's problems are controlled release versions of Sinemet or Madopar, light sedatives and painkillers, or adjustments to his bedding or nightwear. Do discuss these possibilities – and that of aromatherapy – with his GP if you have not already done so.

My friend says that she has been helped a lot by yoga classes. How might this work?

We also know of people who have been helped by yoga. In its overall philosophy and its emphasis on mind over matter, it can give people a sense of purpose and of being in control of their lives. As it can improve people's ability to relax and to keep their joints and muscles mobile and supple, it is easy to see why it might help. It may also improve coordination and relieve some of the muscular aches and pains that are common with Parkinson's. Additionally, the well-being that many people feel after physical activity may help relieve anxiety or any tendency towards depression.

Further information can be obtained from the Yoga for Health Foundation (see Appendix 1 for the address).

Has there been any research into the Alexander Technique and Parkinson's?

The Alexander Technique is a form of complementary therapy using a set of learned mental strategies that concentrate on reducing unnecessary tension. It mainly concentrates on posture, balance and ease of movement – all of which can be affected in Parkinson's. A *randomized clinical trial* showed that it can improve self-assessed disability in people with Parkinson's compared to no intervention or massage. This benefit lasted six months. More research is needed. To find an Alexander Technique teacher near you, contact the Society of Teachers of the Alexander Technique (see Appendix 1 for details).

Does *tai chi* help Parkinson's?

Tai chi promotes a form of moving meditation and is a subtle, gentle exercise that focuses on deep breathing with mental discipline and creative visualization. Physically *tai chi* is a series of coordinated movements, flowing together to become one continuous movement. It increases the body's range of movement, aids relaxation, reduces stress, and assists with good balance and posture.

Two studies in *tai chi* have been reported in the frailty reduction program sponsored by the US National Institute on Aging (NIA). In these studies, the participants (aged 70 or over) improved their walking speed, took more deliberate steps, and had a lower rate of falling. They also reported less fear of falling – and displayed more confidence.

A pilot study on *tai chi* and Parkinson's, at the Redruth Community Hospital, Cornwall, also showed a reduction in falls and the participants reported benefits in walking, sleep and control of their Parkinson's.

The Tai Chi Union for Great Britain and Tai Chi NI (for Northern Ireland) can provide information on classes and instructors (see Appendix 1 for details).

What is acupuncture? Does it have a role in the treatment of Parkinson's?

This ancient form of treatment has been practised in China for over 2000 years. In traditional Chinese medicine it is believed that an energy called *chi* (or *qi*) flows along invisible energy channels called 'meridians', which are linked to internal organs and systems. Inserting fine needles at points along the meridians relating to the affected organ(s) will increase, decrease or unblock the flow of energy. This will stimulate the body's own healing response and help restore natural balance and general well-being.

It is difficult to say whether it has a definite role in the treatment of Parkinson's at the present time. A small *non-blinded* pilot study of the safety, tolerability and efficacy of acupuncture for the symptoms of Parkinson's was recently published. This showed that there were no significant changes in a range of Parkinson's and behavioural symptoms following acupuncture other than in sleep and rest. However, 85% of the participants in the study reported subjective improvement of individual symptoms, including tremor, walking and pain.

Another study is currently looking at the effect of acupuncture on Parkinson's symptoms and quality of life. Further research is needed.

Would reflexology be helpful to someone with Parkinson's?

Reflexology works on the principle that there are reflex areas in the feet (and hands to some extent) which correspond to all the glands, organs and parts of the body. Nerve endings are imbedded in the feet and hands that then travel to the spinal cord and to various parts of the body. Stimulating these nerve endings helps promote relaxation, improves circulation, stimulates vital organs in the body and encourages the body's natural healing processes. The treatment involves light but firm compression massage to the soles and uppers of your feet.

There is a small amount of evidence that supports reflexology but most is still anecdotal rather than based on proper clinical trials. A pilot study on reflexology and Parkinson's is in progress.

There is a lot of publicity about conductive education to help children with *motor disorders* such as cerebral palsy. Has this technique been used to treat people with Parkinson's?

Conductive education is a unique system that incorporates learning on every level – physical, emotional, intellectual and academic. Teachers of conductive education (called conductors) understand that, in order for individuals to develop independence and personal freedom, they must be taught as a whole rather than treated for isolated functions. It aims to help people with motor disorders and neurological conditions to maximize their use of movements, as well as providing techniques for overcoming particular difficulties. Improving self-confidence and developing a positive outlook are also important considerations in conductive education.

There is a large body of *anecdotal evidence* for the benefits of conductive education for people with Parkinson's but research studies so far have been largely flawed, inadequate or inappropriate. Efforts are being made to rectify this and the National Institute for Conductive Education in Birmingham (see Appendix 1) currently has conductive education programmes for people with Parkinson's.

Are there any other complementary therapies that can help in Parkinson's?

There are many other complementary therapies from which people with Parkinson's feel they have benefited. In many cases people benefit because the therapy helps them to relax, or encourages them to exercise or to think positively. Whichever complementary therapy you choose, discuss your ideas with your doctor, check on the therapist's qualifications, and try to talk to other people with Parkinson's who have also tried that particular therapy. It is also a good idea to check what costs will be involved – complementary therapies are not usually available on the NHS and can be quite expensive.

4

Access to treatment and services

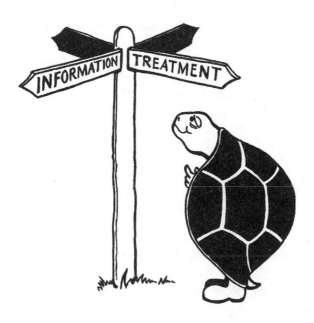

When you need treatment or a particular service, it can be especially frustrating to be passed from pillar to post before discovering the appropriate person or organization. This chapter addresses questions about access to professional services: we hope to make your search for help shorter and more effective. However, we need to add a word of caution. The reorganization of health and social services which began in 1992 is still progressing and this makes it particularly difficult for us to give definite answers to some questions. We will therefore try to outline what we believe to be the general or usual situation, but ask you to refer to organizations in your own local area for details of provision, entitlement and charging.

Medical treatment and related services

How can I find a consultant specializing in Parkinson's?

As Parkinson's is a neurological condition (a condition affecting the body's nervous system), the most appropriate specialist is usually a neurologist. However, not all neurologists specialize in Parkinson's and it is important that you see one who does. As Parkinson's is a condition mainly affecting older people, many geriatricians (doctors specializing in the medical care of older people) are also very knowledgeable about it. To see a specialist, you have to have a referral from your GP who will know if there is a neurologist or geriatrician at your nearest hospital and, if not, where one is located. The Parkinson's Disease Society (see Appendix 1 for address) has a list of consultants with a special interest in Parkinson's and can provide you with details of those working in your area. They are, however, unable to recommend any particular ones.

Are there advantages in making a private appointment?

There may be – if you have private health insurance or if you can otherwise afford it – although the quality of care will not necessarily be better. There is a shortage of neurologists in this country, and as a result some of them have long waiting lists for first appointments and long gaps between follow-up appointments. You still need a referral from your own doctor but, by paying for a private appointment, you may be able to see the specialist more quickly. You can also be sure of seeing that particular person rather than another member of the medical team and you also tend to get rather more time with the specialist.

If money is not a problem, you can remain as a private patient and retain these advantages. However, it is important to remember that treatment is likely to continue for the rest of your life and that the cost may become a very heavy burden. Many specialists will arrange a transfer to their NHS list for people who choose a private first appointment just to obtain a diagnosis and begin treatment.

In some places there are now NHS Parkinson's or neurocare clinics which offer, in addition to medical consultation, access to other members of the health team such as Parkinson's Disease Nurse Specialists, counsellors and therapists. Geriatricians also tend to have access to these other health workers so, in some circumstances, there could be advantages in **not** being a private patient.

What are Patient Advice and Liaison Services (PALS)?

All trusts running hospitals, GP practices or community health services have a Patient Advice and Liaison Service (PALS). These are akin to the customer service desk of the NHS and are designed to offer on the spot help and information such as local health care services and support agencies (including a local branch of the PDS), as well as practical advice and support, with the aim of resolving any problems or difficulties that you may experience while using any NHS services, or if you simply don't know where to turn. PALS also deal informally with concerns expressed (rather than complaints) about all services within the realms of the PCT and send anonymous reports up to the Board of the Trust about what patients are saying about services. The only thing that PALS cannot do is act as an advocate. They don't deal with complaints per se but can tell patients about the NHS complaints system, including details of the local Independent Complaint Advocacy Services (ICAS), which can support people who are making a formal complaint. PALS cannot get involved in a formal complaint.

The PALS service is about giving patients and carers a voice; both in their own care and in the way local health services are run. In order to do this, PALS will record any comments or suggestions you wish to make, and feed them back to the system to ensure that the right lessons are learned and steps taken to tackle problems in order to improve the NHS service.

Your GP surgery or Primary Care Trust should be able to put you in touch with your local PALS.

I would like to see a specialist but my GP refuses to refer me. Can I insist?

There is a widely held belief that you have an absolute right to see a specialist but this is not so. Our understanding is that you have the right to be referred for a second opinion if *you and your GP* agree that this is desirable (our emphasis).

In reality there are things that you can do to increase your chances of being referred. It is helpful to explain fully to your GP why you feel a referral is necessary and to discover the reason for refusal. Usually a GP will think it is reasonable to have the diagnosis and management of Parkinson's confirmed by a specialist. Take a relative or friend with you if you feel that you need moral support or someone to speak for you.

If, having exchanged views, your doctor continues to say 'no' and you still want to pursue the matter, all general practices have an internal complaints system. You would need to talk to the practice manager at your GP surgery to find out how this works. It is important to find out why the referral is being refused, as sometimes lack of neurology services in the area can be a factor.

If this does not resolve the issue, each local authority has procedures for dealing with complaints. The Patient Advice and Liaison Service (PALS) for the Primary Care Trust (PCT) that your GP surgery belongs to should be able to advise you further on any steps that you can take to pursue this further. (See the previous question and a later one on the role of PCTs and PALS). PALS can also put you in touch with the Local Independent Complaints Advocacy Services (ICAS), which can support people who are making a formal complaint. The Patients Association also has a useful booklet called *Making a Complaint* (see Appendix 1 for contact details).

Some people find that changing their GP can solve this problem, as a different one may sometimes be more sympathetic.

However, this cannot be guaranteed, and the pros and cons of such a move need to be carefully considered, especially if, in general, you like your GP and the practice, or it is conveniently situated. Some GP surgeries have closed lists and, if the one you want to change to does, they can refuse you. You then have to apply to the PCT who will allocate you to a GP and it might be that you are allocated to your current one who refused you, or to one that might be less convenient to get to. If you are allocated by the PCT to a GP surgery, they have to accept you. PALS can access information about whether particular GPs have closed books and the allocation process.

Although you have no right to be referred to a specialist, you do have a right to be registered with a GP and to change to another one without giving a reason. Your Primary Care Trust can advise you further about this. (Contact details should be in your local phone book or your GP surgery should be able to provide them. If you have web access, many Primary Care Trusts have websites.)

I have seen a few news items about Parkinson's Disease Nurse Specialists. What are they?

Nurse specialists are a fairly new concept in nursing but they have emerged in several fields in recent years, most notably with the Macmillan Nurses who care for people with cancer. Other nurse specialists work with people who have diabetes, people with asthma, those with bowel and bladder problems and – quite recently, as you note – people with Parkinson's. All nurse specialists have a general nursing training, plus additional qualifications and experience in their chosen specialist field. Parkinson's Disease Nurse Specialists have extensive knowledge about Parkinson's and the drugs used in its treatment, and they work closely with those who have Parkinson's, their carers and other health professionals.

The first Parkinson's Disease Nurse Specialist was appointed in 1989 in Cornwall, and since then, the need for specialist nurses to work with people with Parkinson's and their families has become increasingly apparent. There are currently 120+ Parkinson's

Disease Nurse Specialists employed throughout the UK, who generally work alongside specialists in hospital or in the community working with GPs. They are not yet available in every area but the PDS is actively campaigning for more to be appointed. See the next question for information about how you access them.

How can I get to see a Parkinson's Disease Nurse Specialist?

Contacts with Parkinson's Disease Nurse Specialists are usually at the clinic (Parkinson's, movement disorders, neurological or care of the elderly) or GP's surgery, but they can also do home visits when these are considered necessary. Depending on what other sources of help are available locally, the Parkinson's Disease Nurse Specialist may either concentrate on a particular problem such as drug management, or may be a more general source of advice, support and contact with other services. Access to them varies depending on who employs them and how they work. In many cases, you have to be registered with a doctor that the Parkinson's Disease Nurse Specialist works with, in order to access them. However, in some areas the Parkinson's Disease Nurse Specialist operates a more open access policy. To find out what is available in your area and how you make contact, you should ask your GP or specialist. The PDS helpline can also advise.

Like many new developments, Parkinson's Disease Nurse Specialists are distributed unevenly across the UK, so obtaining access to one is something of a lottery. However, the PDS is committed to increasing the numbers of Parkinson's Disease Nurse Specialists and improving access to them. Contact the PDS community services department for more information on this work.

I have read that exercise and physiotherapy are beneficial but my GP says physiotherapy won't help. What can I do?

To date there have been very few clinical trials that have been undertaken with large enough numbers of people with Parkinson's to prove conclusively the benefits of physiotherapy intervention. This might be what your GP is basing his assumptions on. However, this does not mean that physiotherapy is ineffective, and anecdotally, those who have received input from a physiotherapist have stated that they have been helped in some way. The problem may also lie in what is meant by 'help'. Your GP may mean that physiotherapy cannot cure Parkinson's and, in that, he or she is correct.

However, you are also correct in thinking that, in most cases, exercise and physiotherapy can help by keeping your joints mobile and your muscles supple. Of course the exercise needs to be appropriate for Parkinson's and for you personally. There are also certain strategies you and your family can be taught by the physiotherapist to overcome movement difficulties. Being more mobile and supple will mean that you feel more comfortable, and so more able to keep active and independent.

Most NHS physiotherapy departments have waiting lists, and that may be one reason for your GP's reluctance to make a referral, but some departments do allow *self-referrals* so it would be worth contacting your local hospital or health centre to find out if this is possible. Some local branches of the Parkinson's Disease Society arrange group physiotherapy sessions (see Appendix 1 for the Society's address – they will tell you how to contact your nearest branch), and there are a growing number of private physiotherapists who run clinics and make home visits. If you choose private treatment, you will, of course, have to pay for this yourself, and some physiotherapists may have little experience of treating Parkinson's. You also need to ensure that they are professionally qualified – look for the letters MCSP after their names. This stands for Member of the Chartered Society of Physiotherapists and means that their qualification has been accredited by the Society. However, it could be worth having another discussion with your GP before deciding to start spending money!

You might also like to know that the PDS, working with two physiotherapists, has produced *Keeping Moving*, an exercise video and booklet which contains a programme of exercises for people with Parkinson's to do at home. Contact the PDS for details of cost.

I live in a remote country village and have had Parkinson's for 20 years. I urgently need dental treatment but have severe involuntary movements and can't find a dentist who will accept me. How can I obtain treatment?

Your first move should be to contact your Primary Care Trust (it should be listed in your local phone book) and explain the difficulties you are having. They may know of a dentist who can treat you either in the surgery or at home. A dentist who can offer treatment under sedation (an injection given under the supervision of a doctor after which you remain conscious but relaxed) might be appropriate. If the Primary Care Trust cannot help, you can contact the British Society for Disability and Oral Health (see Appendix 1 for the address and telephone number). They keep a list of dentists interested in treating people with Parkinson's and will try to identify someone for you. Another option might be referral by your dentist or doctor to a dental hospital where inpatient treatment, perhaps under anaesthetic, could be provided.

Living in a remote village is an extra complication but all people with Parkinson's need to take care of their teeth or dentures and to keep their mouths in a healthy condition. This is especially true if they suffer from dryness in the mouth. See the PDS publication *Parkinson's and Dental Health* (B45).

My elderly mother needs her eyes retesting but I don't drive and she is very difficult to move. Could I get someone to come and see her at home?

Yes. Many optometrists will now do home visits. The College of Optometrists has a leaflet *Domiciliary Eye Care Services* which provides advice on what to look for when considering this option. If you have any difficulty finding one who will visit your mother at home, contact your Primary Care Trust who should be able to provide you with a list of local optometrists who do domiciliary eye testing. (The telephone number should be in your local phone book.) If your mother is entitled to a free NHS sight test, this service will be free but otherwise a charge will be made. See the PDS information sheet, *Parkinson's and the Eyes* (FS27).

My speech is becoming less distinct and very hoarse and quiet. I think a speech therapist may be able to help. Can I refer myself or do I need to go through my doctor?

You are wise to consider getting a proper assessment of your speech difficulties and a speech therapist (or *speech and language therapist* as they are now called) is the best person to do this. Although most health districts suffer from a shortage of speech and language therapists, there are a growing number who have an interest in Parkinson's, so you should certainly ask (and if necessary persist in asking) to see one. You can refer yourself by contacting the Speech and Language Therapy Department at your local hospital or health centre, but because of the changing funding arrangements in the NHS, you will have a better chance of getting this service if you get a referral from your GP.

Speech and language therapists can also help with swallowing and drooling problems if these occur.

See the PDS information sheets *Speech and Language Therapy* (FS7) and *Communication* (FS6).

Doing various tasks around the house is becoming more difficult and, as my husband is also disabled, I feel we need some good advice about what to buy, etc. Who could do this?

There are many aids and appliances that can make household tasks more manageable but you are very wise to seek advice first, as it is easy to spend money on things that are not suitable or are unduly expensive. The person who can help is the *occupational therapist*. Your GP, hospital specialist or Parkinson's Disease Nurse Specialist, if you have one, should be able to refer you or you can refer yourself to your local social services department. Some occupational therapists work from a hospital or from Primary Care Trusts and others from social services departments (there is a section on **Primary Care Trusts and social services** later in this chapter).

Sometimes the solution is not a piece of equipment but rather a new way of organizing your work space or of approaching a task, and occupational therapists are very skilled in these matters. The therapist may be able to lend you equipment to try out at home or, alternatively, may arrange a visit to one of the Disabled Living Centres (see Appendix 1 for the Disabled Living Centres Council's address – they will give you details of your nearest centre) where you can see and try some of the bigger and more expensive items.

If the occupational therapist decides that adaptations like rails or ramps are required, then he or she can make a recommendation to the appropriate social services department. There are many variations between areas in the charges made for these aids to daily living and, if you are worried about the possible costs, be sure to mention this to the therapist.

See the PDS information sheet, *Equipment* (FS59) and leaflet on *Occupational Therapy and Parkinson's* (B47).

My walking, even around the house, is not good, but part of the problem is my feet which I am now unable to care for properly. How can I obtain chiropody services?

Comfortable feet are very important for mobility and independence and many people, especially those who are elderly, need access to chiropody (the term podiatry is also used, particularly in English-speaking countries outside the UK) services. People with Parkinson's can be particularly prone to foot problems because of the difficulties that they can experience with walking, posture and foot cramps. They also sometimes have difficulty bending over to cut toenails and generally look after their feet. You should enquire at your GP's surgery about the podiatry services available in your area. Most Primary Care Trusts run clinics and have a domiciliary (home visiting) service for people with mobility problems, so you should be able to arrange regular appointments. It is usually available on the NHS for elderly people and people with physical disabilities that affect their feet or ability to care for their feet.

There are also private podiatrists if you are able to pay. If you do decide to see a podiatrist privately, make sure that he or she is State Registered (they will have the letters SRCh after their name). The Society of Chiropodists and Podiatrists website has a 'find a podiatrist' service as well as useful general information about looking after your feet. (See Appendix 1 for details.)

See the PDS information sheet, *Foot-Care* (FS51).

I know that people with Parkinson's are advised to eat a balanced diet with plenty of fluids and high-fibre foods, but this is difficult for me because of a chronic bowel condition. Could I get some additional advice from a dietitian?

You are quite right about the general dietary advice given to people with Parkinson's (see Chapter 10 for further questions on this topic), but also wise to realize that there can be exceptions to any general rule. First you should talk to your GP or specialist about the ways in which Parkinson's and your bowel condition could affect each other. You could also explain that you want to help yourself by eating sensibly and, if the doctor is not able to offer you enough guidance, you could ask for a referral to a dietitian. Most dietitians work in hospitals but an increasing number are working in the community, and in some places you can approach them directly without going through your GP.

The PDS has two booklets which you might find helpful – *Parkinson's and Diet* (B65) and *Looking after Your Bladder and Bowels in Parkinsonism* (B60).

My elderly father has prostate trouble as well as advanced Parkinson's and is now incontinent at night. Who can I ask for help with the psychological and practical problems this causes?

We assume that everything possible has been done to investigate and treat the incontinence problem. If not, you should contact your father's GP and ask for this to be done as soon as possible. You should also ask his GP to refer him to the local continence adviser or district nurse who will assess his needs and provide advice, support and practical guidance about obtaining pads, pants and laundry services. There is also a confidential advice line run by the Continence Foundation which you can use (see

Appendix 1 for the address and telephone number). Their website also has useful information and a search facility to find continence clinics/advisers in your local area. See also the PDS publication *Looking after Your Bowel and Bladder in Parkinsonism* (B60) which was co-written with the Continence Foundation. A local Parkinson's Disease Nurse Specialist (if available) could also be a useful contact for you. See questions earlier on in this chapter for details of their role.

Primary Care Trusts and social services

I keep hearing the word Primary Care Trusts or PCTs in relation to health services. What are they?

As mentioned in the introduction to this chapter, considerable changes to the NHS are taking place at present. Primary Care Trusts (PCTs) are new local health organizations responsible for managing health services in local areas. They are an integral part of the reorganization of the NHS and will receive 75% of the budget. They work with local authorities and other agencies that provide health and social care locally to make sure the community's needs are being met.

Their responsibilities include making sure there are enough services for people in the area they cover and that these services are accessible. They will ensure that all health services are provided such as GPs, hospitals, dentists, opticians, mental health services, NHS Walk-In Centres, patient transport (including accident and emergency services), population screening, pharmacies and opticians. They are also responsible for getting health and social care systems to work together for the benefit of patients.

There is more information about the reorganization of the NHS on the Department of Health website. (See Appendix 1 for contact details.)

The PDS publication *Meeting Your Health and Social Care Needs* (B70) provides more information on health and social services and how to access them.

Contact details for your local Primary Care Trust should be in your local phone book. If not, your GP surgery should have details. If you have web access, many Primary Care Trusts have their own websites.

What is NHS Direct?

NHS Direct is a telephone patient information service for England and Wales provided by the NHS. It operates a 24-hour nurse advice and health information service, providing confidential information on what to do if you or your family are feeling ill; particular health conditions; local healthcare services, such as doctors, dentists or late night opening pharmacies; and self-help and support organizations. Calls are charged at local rates. A similar service in Scotland, called NHS 24 is being developed. At the time of writing (January 2004), it is only available in some areas but the whole of Scotland should be covered by the end of 2004.

NHS Direct also has a website containing information on a wide range of health issues. (See Appendix 1 for contact details.)

What services do social services departments provide?

Social services departments are part of local authorities and are responsible for providing services to people with various social and welfare needs. People who are elderly or who have a physical, mental or learning disability form the majority of their clients. Social services departments provide (or increasingly nowadays arrange access to) places in luncheon clubs, day centres and *residential homes*; practical help in the home such as *home helps*, *home care workers* and Meals on Wheels; and adaptations and special equipment, which enable people to stay in their own homes. Social services departments also provide information, advice and counselling to people who are old or disabled and to their carers (see Chapter 6 for further discussion of services for carers).

Your local phone book should have contact details of your local social services department. If not, your GP surgery, or Citizens Advice should be able to provide contact details.

My elderly mother is going to come and live with me as she can no longer cope alone. How can I find out what care services are available in my area?

You should contact the social services department and the Primary Care Trust for the area in which you live. They have a duty to provide information about their services and about which people are eligible for them. They can advise on getting an assessment of your mother's needs and should also provide information about any charges which you may incur. The PDS publication *Choices: using and understanding health and social care* (B70) also provides more information. It is important to recognize that, when your mother comes to live with you, you will be her 'carer' and as such are entitled to a care assessment of your own needs. See Chapter 6 *Caring for the 'carers'* – for more information on carers assessments.

What is the difference between home helps and home care workers?

It is difficult to be dogmatic about this and we suspect that there is still considerable overlap between the two roles, but basically home helps assist with general household tasks such as cleaning, cooking and shopping, whereas home care workers tend to concentrate on personal care such as getting washed and dressed (see Chapter 9 for more questions on these topics).

My wife is becoming increasingly disabled with Parkinson's and I have a heart condition. I have been told that we could be eligible for a community care assessment – what does this entail?

Since April 1993 every social services department has been required by law to have a coordinated system for assessing the needs of vulnerable people in the community – a *community care assessment*. In order to request an assessment, all you have to do is to contact your local social services department either directly or through your doctor or other professional worker. (In some areas there is a backlog of assessments, so you may meet delays and some persistence may be required!)

You will then be asked about your needs and, if they cannot be met by the provision of a particular service like home care, but seem rather complex (as they could well be when there are two people with health problems), then an assessor will be assigned to you. He or she will make more detailed enquiries and will coordinate reports from any professionals with relevant knowledge or experience. The aim is to try to fit the services to the client rather than (as often happened in the past) vice versa, and to ensure that you do not have to apply separately to lots of different departments to have your needs assessed.

Two other important characteristics of community care assessments are that the professionals involved are obliged to take account of your views and also to consider (and, if requested, separately assess) the needs of the carer. In your case – and in several others we have encountered – it is not always clear who is caring for whom! If your needs are agreed to be complex and they fall within the criteria established by your social services department, a care manager will be assigned to you (see the answer to the next question for more about care managers).

Every social services department has to publish information about its community care arrangements so you could telephone your local department and ask for a leaflet. These leaflets should also be available in your library, community centre or GP's surgery.

What is a care manager?

A *care manager* is the person from social services or Primary Care Trusts who is given the task of putting together, monitoring and reviewing the plan of care agreed after a community care assessment (discussed in the answer to the previous question).

You should be given a copy of this plan and, if you disagree with what is suggested, your disagreement should be recorded in writing.

If you feel that the plan fails to meet some of your needs, it is important to make this clear and to ask that the plan be reconsidered. Do feel free to involve a relative, friend or voluntary worker, if you are in need of moral or practical support. If none of these people is available to you, ask the social worker or the local Citizens Advice, Council for Voluntary Service (all the addresses and telephone numbers should be in your local phone book) to help you to find an *advocate*, i.e. someone to help you put your point of view.

My mother is nearly blind and my father has Parkinson's. We have asked for a home care worker and someone to help them have a bath but social services say they cannot help. Surely they have to help us?

Without knowing more details, it is difficult for us to judge but it certainly sounds as though you have a case for a proper assessment of your parents' needs (and yours too in so far as you are a carer). Please read the earlier question and answer about community care assessments. If your mother is almost blind and is not registered as blind or partially sighted, arranging such registration through her local social services should improve her access to several services and benefits. Your parents' overall needs will depend on how disabled your father is (people with Parkinson's can be quite capable if their medication is well balanced and they look after themselves in other ways). Home care workers are sometimes forbidden to do housework and, if that is what your parents need, it may be better to try to find someone privately.

The provision of help with bathing from statutory services varies from place to place. In some areas, bathing services are provided by social services, in others by the Primary Care Trust. Another problem arises because of different definitions of 'need'. Your father may feel unable to bathe your mother, even though he is physically capable of doing so, or she may find his help unacceptable. This kind of psychologically or emotionally based need may not be acknowledged by social services as 'real', but if it is a factor in your parents' situation, you should press your case and see if you can get some support from relevant local voluntary organizations who may know of other similar cases.

Adaptations and housing

My mother lives alone but is finding the stairs very difficult to manage. What options does she have to maintain her independence?

There are many different options depending on her wishes, her income, whether the house can be adapted for her needs, and the services available locally from the social services and housing departments.

First you need to sit down with her and discuss what she really wants to do. If her current home is suitable in every aspect except the stairs, then she could decide to live downstairs (if there is space and ground floor toilet and washing facilities) or she could consider having a stairlift installed. She can apply to the social services department to see if she meets their eligibility criteria for this service and, if she does, the social worker will explain when the lift can be supplied (there is sometimes a waiting list) and how much it will cost. The cost will depend on your mother's income. Her chances of being judged eligible for the service will be greater if the provision of a stairlift will substantially improve her chances of retaining her independence. If she is not eligible through social services or if there is likely to be an unacceptably long delay, she could decide to purchase a stairlift herself if she has sufficient funds. Before considering this option, she should get some advice from social services or from an occupational therapist about which makes and models are considered appropriate and whether there is a reputable source of secondhand lifts (which cost much less than new ones). See also the next question on adaptations.

If there seem to be advantages in moving to another house, either to be nearer to sources of help or because her current house has other disadvantages apart from the stairs, she can consider applying for rehousing or selling up and buying a more suitable property. Most areas now have a variety of specialized accommodation for older people offering different levels of supervision and/or support. The local housing department should be able to tell her what is available in the area and what her chances of being allocated certain kinds of accommodation would be. The number for the housing department should be in your local phone book or social services/Citizens Advice should be able to give you the number. The following questions and answers have some more information about this.

Where can I get advice about adapting my home to make it easier for me to manage?

Adaptations can sometimes make life easier and can range from small adaptations, such as grab rails, to major building work, for example to make a home suitable for someone who uses a wheelchair or to put in a downstairs shower and toilet if a person cannot get up stairs.

Before any adaptations are made, it is important to get expert advice. The first person to contact is an occupational therapist who can assess the problems you are having and suggest solutions, which may include adaptations.

Care and Repair, an organization which aims to improve the housing and living conditions of older and disabled people has a useful guide, *In Good Repair*, which gives information on repairs, adaptations, funding and finding a reliable builder or tradesman. This guide will answer most of the questions that enquirers contacting the PDS have. The Disabled Living Foundation and the Centre for Accessible Environments could also advise on the sort of adaptations that might be possible and design issues. See Appendix 1 for contact details.

I own a small terraced house but am finding it difficult to manage. Can I apply to the Council for rehousing?

Yes, you can certainly approach your local authority housing department about any housing problem whether you own your present accommodation or not. The options which will be open to you will depend on the severity of the problems you are facing, local housing resources, the demand for the type of housing you need, and the financial and other conditions that are attached to any such rehousing. However, before thinking of rehousing, check whether your present house could be adapted or some support services provided to help you manage better in your present house. If you would like to do this, contact your local social services department for an assessment of your needs.

We see quite a lot in the papers about sheltered housing. What exactly does it mean and who owns it?

Sheltered housing is accommodation which is purpose-built for people who need a certain amount of supervision because of old age or disability, but who wish to maintain a home of their own. The amount of supervision available can vary from a warden on site who can be contacted in an emergency to high-dependency units where there is still a degree of privacy and independence, but where higher staffing levels allow assistance with meals and personal care. Sheltered housing may be owned by the local authority, by housing associations or by private companies and may be managed by various combinations of these organizations. Your local housing department will be able to provide further information. The number should be in the local phone book. Social services/Citizens Advice should also be able to give you the number.

Questions about residential and nursing homes are discussed in the section on ***Long-term care*** in Chapter 13.

5
Attitudes and relationships

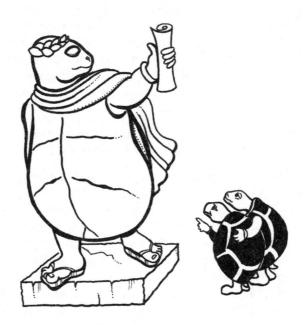

Parkinson's is a real, physical illness. Although it can sometimes be difficult to keep positive, your attitude and approach to managing your condition can make a big difference to how you feel about yourself and how you try to make the best of your life with Parkinson's. This has been emphasized by two people with Parkinson's who have written about their experiences. The first was Sidney Dorros, an American who wrote a book called *Parkinson's: a patient's view*. He liked to talk of 'accommodation without surrender' and would remind people of an old saying – 'If you get a lemon, make lemonade'! The second is a Danish psychologist, Svend Anderson, who has written about his experiences of Parkinson's and the importance of attitude in an information sheet published by the PDS, *The New Role of the Patient* (FS16) and in a book called *Health is Between Your Ears: living with a chronic illness*. See Appendix 2 for details of these books.

This chapter is also about the relationships – family, professional and public – that affect people with Parkinson's and those who live with or look after them. As will become clear, much can depend on the attitudes established in the early weeks and months after diagnosis and on people's willingness to talk through their difficulties and, if necessary, ask for help.

Helping yourself

I have just been diagnosed with Parkinson's. It's a shock but I'd like to think there's something I can do to help myself. Is there?

Yes, there are lots of things you can do and you are already helping yourself by having such a positive attitude. If you think constructively about what you **can** do and how you can avoid and solve problems, you are already giving yourself a very good chance of coping well with Parkinson's. This does not mean that you will feel on top of things every day – none of us do! However, in general, you will be looking for solutions rather than dwelling on problems.

Retaining your interests and activities (or replacing lost ones with something new), learning to maintain a good posture and doing suitable exercises (see Chapters 8 and 9) and eating sensibly (see Chapter 10) are all things that only you can do. Many people are also helped by gathering information about Parkinson's and its treatment (see Chapters 1 to 3), so that they understand better what is happening to them and how things work. Finally, you can continue as you have started by being willing to ask questions and so being really involved in planning your own care.

There are also some commercially published books by people with Parkinson's that promote a positive attitude. These include those by Sidney Dorros and Svend Andersen mentioned at the beginning of this chapter, *Lucky Man* by Michael J. Fox and *Living Well with Parkinson's* by Glenna Wooton Atwood. See Appendix 2 for details.

You and your partner

I have just been diagnosed and don't want to tell my wife and family. What do you think I should do?

As we don't know you or the other members of your family, we can't give you specific advice but we can offer some ideas and questions for you to consider.

First you could try thinking through the consequences of telling or not telling your wife and family. If they know that you have been having some problems and that you have consulted the doctor, they will be expecting some information about the outcome. They will also have their own thoughts and fears, and you will not know whether these are more or less distressing than a diagnosis of Parkinson's. Even quite small children can sense when something is wrong, and pretending otherwise will not necessarily reassure them.

The other problem with not telling the truth is that the secret can come between you and your loved ones, creating barriers where there were none before. You may also be depriving yourself of a very important source of help and comfort. However, you may have some special reason for not 'telling' just yet, either because you are not feeling ready to talk about it or because one or more of your family are having some difficulties of their own just now.

It might be worth you talking the pros and cons over with a friend or counsellor. If you have no obvious source of help available locally, you could perhaps try the Parkinson's Disease Society's Helpline (see Appendix 1 for the phone number). You will have to weigh the arguments for and against telling your wife and family, but do remember that the task may seem to get bigger the longer you leave it.

I am 47, divorced but have a wonderful girlfriend. We had planned to marry but I have now been told I have Parkinson's. I don't know whether to go ahead with our plans or not.

If you have read Chapters 1 and 2 of this book you will know just how variable the impact of Parkinson's can be and how impossible it is to know what the future holds for any one individual. We do know that, with the current treatments available, life expectancy is not very different for people with Parkinson's from the normal life expectancy. Many people cope well and have satisfying lives for many years.

Parkinson's is a factor that you need to think about when considering your future with your girlfriend and each couple's response to Parkinson's will be different. Clearly you will have to talk to your girlfriend and you will both need to be honest about how you feel. It is important to explore any aspects of Parkinson's that either of you have particular concerns about before making a decision.

You could perhaps go together to speak to your neurologist or GP. Friends or relatives could perhaps provide individual opportunities for you both to mull things over with a sympathetic listener. Alternatives might be your local branch of Relate or the Parkinson's Disease Society's Helpline. As you are 47 you might also find it helpful to have contact with the PDS's special interest group for younger people with Parkinson, YAPP&RS (Young Alert Parkinson's Partners and Relatives). See Appendix 1 for contact details.

It may reassure you to know, however, that the PDS knows several couples who met and married after one of them was diagnosed with Parkinson's, who have managed very well and are very happy.

My husband, diagnosed earlier this year, gets tired easily. Should I encourage him to rest as much as possible?

Although it is true that fatigue is a common and often under-estimated symptom of Parkinson's, it is also important that your husband keeps as active and involved in things as possible. If he becomes more dependent on you than is necessary, he will tend to feel helpless and bored, will have fewer topics to talk about and may become more liable to depression. In addition you will become more tied to the house and less able to keep up your own activities and interests, so both of you will suffer. The PDS has an information sheet on *Fatigue* (FS72), which you might find helpful. We would also suggest that your husband discusses the tiredness with his doctor or Parkinson's Disease Nurse Specialist who might be able to advise further. Tiredness can also sometimes be the symptom of other health problems, including depression, which is common in Parkinson's, so it is important to check.

One possible solution is to encourage your husband to pace himself, doing things for himself at times when he is at his best and taking rests as necessary. If he rests too much during the day, his sleep at night may be affected, so creating another problem.

One of the big difficulties for relatives of people with Parkinson's is knowing when to encourage them to do things for themselves and how to recognize the times when this is not possible. As abilities can vary from day to day – and even from hour to hour – this is not easy and requires great patience and sensitivity. Try to get other family members to understand how to keep this balance too. Don't be too discouraged if you don't always get it right. It **is** difficult and people don't become saints just because they or their spouses develop Parkinson's!

I'm a hyperactive, rather impatient person and I'm feeling really bad about the way I snap at my wife who has Parkinson's and is therefore slower than she used to be. What can I do to make things easier for both of us?

Your question is a courageous and honest effort to face up to a difficult problem. As indicated in the answer to the previous question, people who develop Parkinson's, and their partners and families, do not stop being the people they were before. The challenge is to find a new way of living which takes account of all the elements in the new situation.

Perhaps the best way for you and your wife to start is to sit down together and acknowledge the problem and your sadness that you sometimes hurt each other. If you think her slowness has got worse recently, you could check with her GP or consultant whether any adjustment to her medication might help. Meanwhile you can try to identify the particular situations that you both find most frustrating and plan ways of avoiding or easing them. You may not realize, for example, that trying to hurry people with Parkinson's can make them slower, not faster. Both of you need to allow plenty of time for the tasks you intend to tackle, so you have to accept the need for much more planning in your lives. One person with Parkinson's told us that this was, for him, the hardest thing to accept, so we are not suggesting that it is easy! Having allowed enough time (and, where possible, having programmed activities for a part of the day when your wife is at her best), don't stand around and watch while your wife gets dressed etc., unless she needs your active assistance – go and do something else!

An extension to this last point is that you both need to retain or acquire some enjoyable activities that you can pursue independently of each other. Then, when you are together, you may find that you are able to be more relaxed and patient. For information about longer breaks, see Chapter 13.

You might also get some benefit from meeting other carers and discovering that other people have similar feelings and problems. Your local PDS branch will provide opportunities for you to meet other carers and there may also be a local carers support group or centre run by carers organizations such as Carers UK and Princess Royal Trust for Carers. See Appendix 1 for contact details.

We have a very happy marriage, perhaps partly because we've always had some individual as well as shared interests. Now my husband has got Parkinson's and I'm afraid I will resent having to give up my own 'space'. Am I being selfish?

Your fears are very understandable and probably not selfish at all. Most doctors and other professionals involved with people who have been recently diagnosed, stress the need for both parties to maintain their interests and independence and to live as normal a life as possible. Because Parkinson's can be difficult to diagnose, some people have been through many months of anxiety and uncertainty by the time that they get the diagnosis and treatment can begin. This can mean that they have already withdrawn a bit from their activities and their partner has had to do the same. However, once your husband has the correct treatment, you should both be able to pick up all or most of your earlier interests. As you suggest, such diversity can actually strengthen a marriage and it can certainly make any necessary adjustments which follow the onset of Parkinson's easier to handle.

I don't know how much longer I can cope. My husband was the dominant, decision-making partner in our marriage and we both liked it that way. Now he is quite disabled with Parkinson's but the real problem is that we don't seem to be able to adjust to our new roles – I feel over-whelmed and indecisive. He feels frustrated and angry.

Every marriage or relationship is unique and there are many different ways of sharing the roles and being happy. The problems arise, as you have discovered, when circumstances change and your particular solution no longer works. We can't tell from your question whether you have felt able to sit down and talk these matters over with your husband. If you haven't, that would be the place to start. Outside help – from a trusted friend, from the PDS, a carers organization such as Carers UK and Princess Royal Trust for Carers, or a counsellor working at Relate may also enable you both to explore whether the situation can be improved and, if so, how. See Appendix 1 for contact details.

**I am 36, have recently been diagnosed as having
Parkinson's and am beginning to understand some of the
symptoms and also what can be done to help. The thing
that worries me most is how it might affect my
relationship with my husband.**

This is a very understandable concern and it is a good sign that
you can put your anxieties into words. Perhaps you will be able
to take the next step and talk it over with your husband – you will
probably find that he has some anxieties about this too.

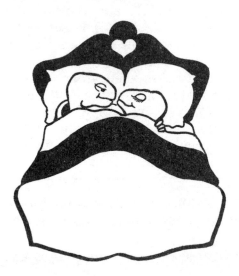

'Relationships' within marriage have many features including
the way in which roles are shared as well as specific emotional
and sexual aspects. Almost everything that happens to a couple
can affect their emotional and sexual relationships, and there is
no doubt that Parkinson's can call for quite a lot of adjustments.
There are very close links between how people feel about
themselves and how satisfied they feel with their marital/sexual
relationships. Any illness or disability can affect our self-image
and our most intimate relationships. However, it is also true that
many people continue to have satisfactory marital and sexual
relationships despite having Parkinson's.

If it is the sexual aspects which cause you particular concern, The PDS booklet *Sex and Intimate Relationships* (B34) may be useful to you. It includes information on how Parkinson's may affect sexual relationships as well as treatments that are available to help. From research undertaken into sexual relationships and Parkinson's, stress, anxiety and depression seemed to be more important causes of problems than anything directly related to the Parkinson's, and something can usually be done to help in such circumstances.

One important piece of advice offered by several people with Parkinson's is to retain and treasure the small signs of affection and togetherness – touches, cuddles, kisses – which remind both the person with Parkinson's and the carer that they are loveable and loved. If you do not already know about YAPP&RS, the special Parkinson's Disease Society group for younger people like yourself, you can find information about it in Chapter 15. You might find it helpful to discuss some of your fears with others who are in a similar position. Your consultant or Parkinson's Disease Nurse Specialist might also be able to help. See Appendix 1 for contact details.

Does Parkinson's cause impotence? My husband has become impotent at the age of 39, four years after being diagnosed.

Parkinson's can cause erectile dysfunction (the preferred term used by doctors to describe *impotence*) as can the stress and anxiety which are sometimes associated with it. Some drugs used for other conditions, including some of the new antidepressants, may also have this side effect. If your husband has not already sought help, you should talk to him about the problem and encourage him to do so. His GP or neurologist may be able to help by referring him to someone with special expertise in this field.

Emotional support and counselling may be enough but, if not, there are other options which can be tried. These include the much publicized drug Viagra (generic name sildenafil), Yohimbine tablets, a vacuum pump, and injection of a drug called papaverine directly into the penis. The availability of these treatments on the NHS seems to vary depending on local arrangements, so it is important to explore what is available where you live. In the case of Viagra, Parkinson's is included on the list of conditions that can cause erectile dysfunction and can be treated with this drug on the NHS.

Does Parkinson's have any effect on fertility?

For obvious reasons, the number of people with Parkinson's who are at the childbearing stage of life is very small, but we know of both men and women with Parkinson's who have produced children after they have been diagnosed.

Children and grandchildren

I am 38 and was recently diagnosed with Parkinson's. The treatment is working well and only a few tell-tale symptoms remain. We have two young children aged 6 and 4 and my wife and I can't decide what to tell them. What do you think?

Obviously your children are too small for complicated explanations but, as in our answers in the previous section about the pros and cons of telling family members, we think that honesty is usually the best policy. With small children, who can be very sensitive to anxiety in their parents, you can just answer their questions as they arise or explain simply why you are tired or unsteady or whatever.

There is a booklet for young children (*Gramps/Grandma has PD*), produced by the Parkinson's Disease Society in English, Urdu, Gujerati, Punjabi, and a special version for Afro-Caribbean families – it addresses the more common situation of grandparents with Parkinson's. However, it may give you some ideas about how to talk to your small children. There is also a story book, suitable for children aged roughly between 3 and 12

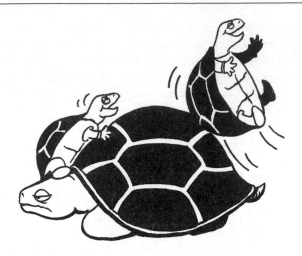

years, called *Our Mum has Parkinson's*, told from the viewpoint of an 11-year-old girl and written by a teacher who has Parkinson's. The PDS also publishes an information sheet, *Talking to Your Children about Parkinson's* (FS66), which you might find helpful.

You could also talk to your children's teachers to see if there is any help that they can provide. Some people say that their children have found it helpful to take one of the booklets described in the previous paragraph to school for 'show and tell' times.

As you are only 38, you might also find it helpful to make contact with the PDS's group for younger people with Parkinson's, YAPP&Rs. There are likely to be other people with children who can offer mutual support.

My husband has had Parkinson's for nearly 20 years and is now quite disabled but he does love to have our grandchildren come to visit. However, most of them live some distance away and can be quite daunted by his appearance and his mobility problems. What can we do to make their visits easier and more enjoyable for everyone?

You can encourage your children to visit with the grandchildren at times when your husband is likely to be at his best and therefore more able to talk and listen and play. When his medication is working most effectively, his expression and mobility are likely to be less daunting to the grandchildren. A bit of explanation beforehand to the children about granddad's illness and the way that it hides 'the real granddad' may also help. See also the publications mentioned in the previous answer. Try to think of enjoyable and novel things to do while they are with you but do not allow the visits to be overlong. If your children or grandchildren want to help in some way, let them. Most of us feel more comfortable when we are being useful. Some of the publications mentioned in the previous question might also be helpful.

My husband has had Parkinson's for many years but we have managed to keep up a normal family life and the children have taken the few necessary adjustments in their stride. Now one son is 14 and discipline is becoming a problem. Some of the rows have been particularly hurtful to my husband. Is there anything we can do to improve matters?

Coping with adolescence creates problems for most families and there are no easy answers. You may find that talking things over with other couples, who are not also coping with a disabling illness, helps to put things in perspective. You need to explore why he is causing such disruption. Is there something that is particularly bothering him? Is it related to your husband's Parkinson's? If so, the PDS publication, *Talking to Your Children about Parkinson's* (FS66) for parents like yourselves, might be helpful.

Talking among yourselves, acknowledging feelings on all sides and exploring how to avoid or cope better with the 'trigger' situations may also help. You may want to consider contacting YAPP&RS, the special section of the Parkinson's Disease Society for younger people. There are sure to be people there who have experienced similar problems who might be able to offer some suggestions.

If none of this seems sufficient, you could speak to the confidential Helpline at the Parkinson's Disease Society (address and telephone number in Appendix 1). You might also find that there is a sympathetic teacher or educational counsellor at his school who might be able to provide you with some advice.

Outside the family

When my doctor sent me to see the consultant neurologist and Parkinson's was diagnosed, he explained quite well but seemed to imply that I was lucky it was Parkinson's. I don't feel at all lucky – how could he think that?

You have touched on an important topic which can lead to mutual misunderstanding between doctors and their patients, so it is helpful for us to have an opportunity to try and unravel the issues. One of the most powerful influences on our satisfaction or dissatisfaction with things that happen to us is what we are expecting, and that in turn depends in part on our previous experiences. This is true whether we are talking about our reactions to an evening out or to the news that we have a medical condition like Parkinson's.

The experiences of medically-trained people like neurologists and their non-medical patients are very different. Without knowing what you thought the cause of your problem might be, it's difficult to guess your first reaction to the diagnosis but, if you did feel as shocked and dismayed as your question suggests, you would not be unusual. There is no doubt that there are lots of disadvantages to having Parkinson's including the fact that, although treatment is available, there is as yet no cure.

A possible clue to your impression that the neurologist thought you were lucky can be found in that last sentence. Neurologists deal mainly with conditions for which, like Parkinson's, there is presently no cure, but for many of the other conditions there is no effective treatment either. In some conditions (**not** Parkinson's) the life expectation after diagnosis may be quite limited. So if you can imagine yourself in the neurologist's place, knowing all that they know, then you can perhaps see why they feel much better about giving a diagnosis for which some treatment and the hope of improvement especially in the short and medium term can be offered.

However, understanding how such attitudes can arise does not mean that they should be encouraged. If we want to establish trust between people with Parkinson's and doctors, in order to work well together over many years after diagnosis, then doctors need guidance about how to give the diagnosis. How to develop an attitude to Parkinson's which is both honest and hopeful and which also acknowledges people's fears and uncertainties is important. It is no help when you are grieving about breaking one leg to be told that you are lucky not to have broken two! When you can think like this, you know that you are beginning to come to terms with what has happened.

I find it difficult to talk to my doctor. Do you have any tips?

The PDS has an information sheet, *Tips for Talking to Your Doctor* (FS71), which contains suggestions such as those highlighted below and useful resources. The PDS Helpline can also discuss any particular difficulties that you have with talking to your doctor. (See Appendix 1 for contact details.)

- Make a list of the concerns that you want to discuss with the doctor – keep them brief and specific as possible and put the most important questions at the top. If you find it hard to ask the doctor the questions on the list or find it hard to communicate, give the list to the doctor when you have your appointment.

- Keeping a weekly or monthly diary of how you have managed your symptoms can be useful. The PDS publishes two information sheets with sample diaries, *Keeping a Diary – people with Parkinson's* (FS69) and *Keeping a Diary – carers* (FS70), which you might find useful.

- Take with you any tablets that you are taking (in the bottle or packaging). This is important because people with

Parkinson's are often on complicated drug regimens involving several different types of tablets. It can be hard to remember the names of each one. GPs we consulted said that they found it much easier to discuss the tablets if their patients showed them the bottles or packets of tablets rather than referring to 'small white ones' or 'the ones I take at night.'

- If you have several problems to discuss, it may be best to make separate appointments or ask for a double appointment.

- Take someone with you – to give you moral support, act as an advocate or help you remember what was said and take notes.

- Be honest. Many people feel they have to put their best face on for the doctor and show them how well they are coping when the reality is quite different. The doctor can only give you the best treatment if you tell them what is really happening to you.

- Don't be afraid to ask questions. If you are going to get the best from your treatment you need to make sure that you understand what you need to do. Get your partner or friend to take notes if it helps. If they use technical language or medical jargon to describe symptoms or treatment and you don't understand, ask them to explain it to you.

- Many people find it hard to talk about embarrassing subjects – tell the doctor if you do find it hard but make sure you do talk to them about anything that is important to you. You won't be the first person to ask!

- Keep informed – if you understand your Parkinson's, you will find it easier to cope, discuss your care with your doctor and make decisions about your care.

I work with a man who has Parkinson's. He is good at his job but seems very reserved and isolated. I don't want to intrude but wonder if I should encourage him to get more involved with other people at work?

Although people with Parkinson's are as diverse as anyone else in their personalities and attitudes, there are some aspects of the condition which make those who have it especially prone to isolation. If you are aware of these aspects, you will perhaps be able to explore them tactfully with your colleague and so discover whether his reserve is real and his isolation freely chosen. The PDS has information and tips to help people like yourself communicate with people with Parkinson's. If he would like to be more sociable, it will be helpful for him to have your understanding and practical support.

The first thing to realize is that the rigidity of muscles in Parkinson's interferes with spontaneous movements and that it can lead to a 'mask-like' expression which makes smiling and showing interest more difficult. In these cases you might assume that someone is uninterested or bored when that is not the case at all.

On the other hand, people with Parkinson's sometimes withdraw from social contacts because they feel embarrassed by symptoms such as slowness, tremor or speech problems. If they can be helped to feel accepted and understood and given time to join in the conversation, they can become more confident again.

Finally, people with Parkinson's do tend to suffer from fatigue and, if they are doing a full-time job, this is especially likely. It may therefore be that your colleague has made a conscious decision to conserve his energies for work rather than socializing.

I manage to keep quite active in spite of having Parkinson's for more than five years. However, my walking is rather unsteady and passers-by sometimes stare or make comments as though I was drunk. It's very hurtful. How can we help people become more understanding?

We sympathize with your feelings of hurt about your experience, which is not that uncommon. With regard to your walking, have you seen a physiotherapist as they would be able to assess your walking and give you advice that might make it easier? You are right, however, to focus on what we can do about it. Really it comes down to education – everything from public awareness campaigns and media coverage to information for individuals. The Parkinson's Disease Society (see Chapter 15 for more information) is constantly trying to devise ways of raising public awareness, but there may be things that you could do yourself. If you felt able to do so, you could stop and say that you have Parkinson's or perhaps show an Alert Card (one available from the Parkinson's Disease Society is shown in Figure 5.1), which explains that you have a neurological condition which affects your walking and balance. Every little helps.

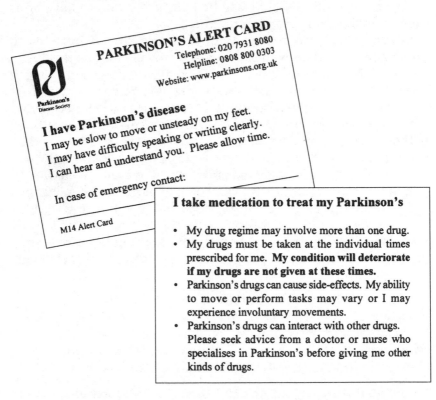

Figure 5.1 Alert Card produced by the Parkinson's Disease Society

6
Caring for the 'carers'

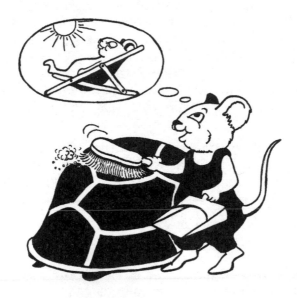

Partners, relatives and friends of people with Parkinson's 'live' with Parkinson's too. If this describes you, how Parkinson's affects your life will depend very much on many factors, such as your individual circumstances, the symptoms the person you are close to has, the specific help they need, and your relationship with them. This chapter aims to address some of the questions that you may have.

In this book, we have sometimes used the word 'carer', which is a term used to describe anyone of any age who cares on an informal basis for someone close to them who, because of illness, disability or frailty, needs support. The type of support given varies enormously. In the case of Parkinson's, many people cope very well with the condition without requiring a lot of looking after. However, sometimes people do need considerable practical and emotional support. Whatever the situation, if you are a carer, it is important to remember that you need information and advice to help you cope. If you are finding it difficult to manage, remember that support is available to help you. We describe some of the services in this chapter. More information can be obtained from the PDS resources for carers, which include *The Guide* (B71) and videos, *No More Secrets* (V7) for new carers and *The Long-Term Carers Companion: an A-Z guide* (V9). Contact the PDS for details of costs.

You may also find it helpful to read also Chapter 5 on **Attitudes and Relationships**, Chapter 7 on **Communication** and Chapter 13 **Care Outside the Home** in this book.

I have lived all my life with my mother who has Parkinson's and we are good friends as well as mother and daughter. I suppose that I am her 'carer' but I don't really like the word.

We understand your feelings about this word and your difficulty in applying it to yourself. In fact most of us resent being reduced to any one 'label' and fight to retain our own individual sense of ourselves. However, the increased use of the word 'carer' has coincided with a growing awareness, among professionals and the general public, of the needs of people like yourself. Parkinson's usually lasts for many years and, however good the relationship, it can bring limitations to the person who is caring as well as to the person with Parkinson's. Recognizing and valuing carers is important to ensure that support is available to help them cope, for instance financial support or providing respite care occasionally to allow carers to have time to themselves to follow their own interests and recharge their batteries.

Our message would therefore be – yes, you are much more than a carer, but don't let that fact stop you from taking advantage of any emotional, practical or financial help available, which is discussed in some of the following questions.

I have been looking after my wife for 22 years. Mostly I don't mind the work or the responsibility but I do hate being taken for granted. Just occasionally I would like someone to ask about me.

We are sure that your words sum up the feelings of many people who look after their spouses or other relatives. In fact, when a group of people caring for their Parkinson's relatives got together with the PDS to discuss their needs, recognition and acknowledgment were at the top of their list. To be told that you are doing a good job, to be asked for your opinion or to receive a caring enquiry about your own health and spirits can be a real boost.

Quite a lot of training for doctors, nurses, therapists and home carers is now including this sort of message, and many educators are discovering that the best people to deliver the message are people like yourself, who know what it is like to be a carer, 24 hours a day, 7 days a week.

Since you have been caring for your wife for 22 years, we imagine that your caring role may be a considerable one by now. Are there aspects of this that are causing you concern or where you could do with some extra help? An assessment of your needs and your wife's through social services might be helpful. This would give you an opportunity to discuss your role as a carer and identify services, such as respite care, to provide you with support. See the question on carers' assessment later on in this chapter for more details.

Is your own health causing you some concern? If so, it might be a good idea to have a check-up with the doctor. Carers often neglect themselves because they are so busy looking after their partner or relative but, in the long run, it is much better for both parties if the carer's health is also a priority.

The PDS resources for carers, mentioned at the beginning of this chapter, might be useful to you. You might also find it helpful to talk to other carers to provide mutual support and exchange ideas. You can meet others through a local PDS branch or carers' organization such as Carers UK and The Princess Royal Trust for Carers (see Appendix 1 for details). These organizations could also provide you with information and support.

I am 55, fit and competent and very happy to care for my husband who is older than I am and who has had Parkinson's for many years. What riles me is the struggle to obtain proper information about the services and benefits that are available – I can spend hours on the phone trying to locate the right office or person.

You are right to identify accurate and accessible information as a prime need of carers and to underline the stress and frustration that you experience when it is not available. It is unfortunately the case that, in some instances, what should be easily available in fact requires great persistence! The PDS can advise you further on services and benefits. You might also find the resources mentioned at the beginning of this chapter helpful. Carers' organizations such as Carers UK and The Princess Royal Trust for Carers can also provide information and advice. For instance, Carers UK (see Appendix 1 for their address) has, in addition to its national literature, helped to produce information guides called the *Carers' A to Z* in many different parts of the country. Ask at your local social services, library or health centre to discover whether there is one for your area. Princess Royal Trust for Carers has carers' centres in many parts of the country where you can get advice and support. (See Appendix 1 for contact details.)

Access to information should also be improving in all areas as a result of the Community Care Act, the Carers Act 1995 and the government's announcement in early 1999 of a new deal for carers. These various measures mean that social services departments have to provide information about the services available in their locality, take account of the needs of carers when carrying out community care assessments, and provide better access to *respite care*. Also, under the Carers and Disabled Children Act 2000, carers now have the right to an assessment regardless of whether the person they care for is having their needs assessed. As a result of this, the carer can have services provided just for them (see next question for more information). The government has also developed a carers website – www.carers.gov.uk – to help provide more information. Some social services departments and Primary Care Trusts also have carers workers.

With respect to financial benefits, the PDS has a Welfare and Employment Rights Department, which produces a number of information sheets on finance and employment for people with Parkinson's and their carers. See also the PDS publication *Choices: using and understanding health and social care* (B70), *Carers Assessment* information sheet (FS46) and Chapter 4 of this book for information about obtaining access to a wide range of treatments and services).

Who is entitled to a separate carer's assessment?

A carer is anyone who helps to look after another person, such as a spouse or partner, relative, friend or neighbour, and who provides a substantial amount of regular care. With the introduction of the Carers' Recognition and Services Act 1995, the government formally recognized, for the first time, the valuable contribution of carers to the provision of care in the community and acknowledged that community care depends on carers.

If the person being cared for is being assessed, their carer has the right to be assessed for his/her needs too. In addition, under the Carers and Disabled Children Act 2000, carers now have the right to an assessment regardless of whether the person they care for is having their needs assessed. As a result of this, the carer can have services provided just for them. The services can include respite care, emotional support from other carers, help with caring and household tasks, and activities for the person cared for. However, no new money has been allocated to local authorities to aid the Act's implementation. Therefore how this works depends on the funding situation in a particular local authority. What is available and who pays for it can vary considerably between different authorities.

If you want to arrange a carer's assessment, you need to contact your local social services department. Further information on carers' assessments is available from the PDS, Carers UK and the Princess Royal Trust for Carers (see Appendix 1 for contact details).

My wife is now very disabled and can't turn over or get in and out of bed without help. I am exhausted and feel in need of a rest. Could we get a night sitter?

Sleep and night-time problems are common for people with Parkinson's and carers. The PDS has an information sheet, *Sleep and Night-time Problems* (FS30), written by a Parkinson's specialist, which you might find helpful. Night-time problems can sometimes be eased by changes in medication. If you have not already discussed this with your wife's doctor, we would urge you to do so. A physiotherapist and/or an occupational therapist can also help with practical advice for both the person with Parkinson's and their carer (see Chapter 9 for further discussion of this topic). Do ask your GP for a referral if you have not had access to such advice before. See Chapter 4 *Access to treatment and services* for more information on what these professionals do.

One practical tip, if turning over in bed is a particular problem for your wife, is that some people find satin or silky sheets or wearing satin or silky nightwear can make this easier.

Some Primary Care Trusts and social services departments have a night sitting service, although it is often pretty limited. Your GP should be able to advise further. Private sitters are also available but tend to be rather costly and you need to be sure that they are reputable. Again your GP or Primary Care Trust should have some information. The UK Home Care Association (UKHCA) might also be able to advise (see Appendix 1 for contact details).

There are other ways of arranging some respite for yourself and you will find examples of these in the answer to the next question and in Chapter 13 on *Care outside the home*.

My 80-year-old mother is now very frail and requires constant supervision. I am single and have no brothers or sisters, so I feel trapped in the house and more and more stressed. Can you suggest any solution?

All carers need some time for themselves if they are to continue being able to care, and you have obviously tried to manage without such help for too long. Approach your social services department and ask them to assess your needs as a carer (as well as your mother's) and say that you need regular respite care for your mother. See the question on carers' assessment that appears earlier on in this chapter for more details.

There are a number of ways that respite care can be provided. These include someone coming in to stay with your mother once or twice a week, day centres, or care provided away from home to allow the carer to have a short or long break. Some social services departments now have contracts with Crossroads – Caring for Carers, an organization whose objective is to give people like you a break. If you have a local Crossroads scheme, you could also approach them direct (see your phone book for a local number, or see Appendix 1 for contact details for the national organizations). The local PDS Branch might also be able advise on what is available in your area.

My wife is now very immobile and I often have to ask our teenage daughter to help me lift her or to stay in while I am working late. She is devoted to her mother but I don't want to take away her youth. How can I balance all our needs?

This is a difficult and sensitive problem. If you are convinced that everything possible has been done to maximize your wife's mobility, then you need to sit down together and discuss what options you have for rearranging your daily and weekly routines. Much will depend on what kind and quantity of help, from family and friends or from statutory and voluntary services, is available to you.

It sounds as though a thorough, *multidisciplinary assessment* (involving medical, nursing, therapy and social services personnel) would help, and you can request this through your GP or social services department. There is now much more awareness of the needs of carers, including young carers, than there was. If your wife's needs are being assessed, you and your daughter as carers have the right to have your needs assessed too. Also under the Carers and Disabled Children Act 2000, carers have the right to an assessment regardless of whether the person they care for is having their needs assessed. This includes children and teenagers who help with care tasks. As a result, the carer can have services provided just for them. See the PDS booklet *Meeting Your Health and Social Care Needs* (B70) and information sheet *Carers Assessments* (FS46) for more information

It is certainly wise to ensure that your daughter is able to spend time with her friends and to have leisure activities suited to her age, but she may also enjoy, and benefit from, the time she spends with her mother and feel good about being able to help. You don't say whether you also have a son. If you do, you should try to share the caring tasks between them rather than assume that these are girls' jobs. Most people find some caring tasks easier to cope with than others. It would be worth trying to discover if there are tasks such as toileting or bathing which your daughter or your wife find particularly distressing. You could then feed this information into the assessment process.

You do not say if your daughter is still at school. It might be a good idea to discuss her caring role with her school, as it may have an effect on her ability to cope with her studies.

Several organizations, including Carers UK, the Princess Royal Trust for Carers, the Children's Society and some Crossroads – Caring for Carers schemes provide information and support to young carers. See Appendix 1 for contact details.

My wife has had Parkinson's for over 20 years and I have no problems coping with the physical tasks of caring. However, she has recently become quite confused and sometimes does not recognize me. I find this very distressing and would appreciate some practical and emotional support.

Support for the carers of people suffering from confusion and dementia (the general name for an illness in which the brain cells die faster than they do in normal ageing) is absolutely essential because, as you say, it is so distressing. However, first you must ensure that your wife's new symptoms are not due to some other temporary cause like infection, medicines or some other illness, so ask your doctor about this as soon as possible.

If the doctor decides that the cause of your wife's deteriorating mental abilities is dementia, organizations like the Alzheimer's Society and Alzheimer's Scotland – Action on Dementia, can provide you with information, practical advice and emotional support. They support people with all kinds of dementia and their families.

You might get support from other people coping with similar problems through a local Alzheimer's group, PDS branch or carers group. You can also apply to the social services department (see your local phone book for their number) for an assessment of your wife's needs and your needs as carer. They will then be able to propose a package of services to meet your needs (see Chapter 4 for more information about these community care assessments).

There are also some very helpful booklets for carers of people suffering from confusion and dementia. These include *Coping with Dementia: a handbook for carers* available from Alzheimer's Scotland and *Caring for Someone with Dementia* published by Age Concern (see Appendix 2 for details). The PDS also has an information sheet on *Dementia* (FS58), which includes information on communicating with someone with dementia.

My husband has had Parkinson's for the last six years but he has also developed some serious mental and behavioural problems and is not recognizable as the man I married. He keeps exposing himself and trying to touch any female who comes to the house. The result is that my friends are embarrassed to call and I am losing my friends as well as my husband. Please help!

This is an extremely difficult problem. Inappropriate behaviour such as this can be a side effect of the Parkinson's drugs, general mental deterioration which may or may not be due to Parkinson's, or frustration – or a combination of all three. If you have not already sought any help, it is important that you discuss this with your GP and Parkinson's specialist. Depending on his or her overall view of your husband's condition, a referral can be made to another specialist such as a psychiatrist. The PDS booklet *Sex and Intimate Relationships* (B34) contains a section on drug-side effects such as these.

You could try to screw up the courage to confide in your closest friends and see if they feel able to share the problem with you rather than hide away from it. It will help if you can reassure them that he really means no harm and is not fully responsible for his actions.

The other thing that will help is for you to have some days when you are not responsible for his care. You could try to arrange some day care through the social services department or hospital and, while he is away, try to get out and do something which you enjoy.

I am the 'carer' for my husband at present, but he would like very much to be more in control of what he does. I have heard of the Expert Patient Programme run by the NHS, but what exactly is it?

The Expert Patient Programme (EPP) is an NHS-based training programme that provides opportunities for people who live with long-term chronic conditions to develop new skills to manage their condition better on a day-to-day basis. Set up in April 2002, it is based on research from the US and UK over the last two decades, which shows that people living with chronic illnesses are often in the best position to know what they need in managing their own condition. Provided with the necessary 'self-management' skills, they can make a considerable impact on the management of their condition and their quality of life.

'Expert Patients' are defined by the NHS as 'people living with a long-term health condition, who are able to take more control over their health by understanding and managing their conditions, leading to an improved quality of life.' Expert patients:

- feel confident and in control of their lives

- aim to manage their condition and its treatment in partnership with healthcare professionals

- communicate effectively with professionals and are willing to share responsibility on treatment

- are realistic about the impact of their disease on themselves and their family

- use their skills and knowledge to lead full lives.

Becoming an expert patient involves taking a 6-week course lasting 2½ hours per week led by people who live with a long-term health condition.

For more information about courses in your area, you can contact their enquiry line on 0845 606 6040 or website – www.expertpatients.nhs.uk.

7
Communication

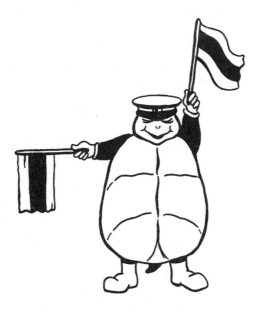

The questions in this chapter are about *communication*. People with Parkinson's often find all kinds of communication are limited by the Parkinson's symptoms. Not just about *speech*, which is only one of the many ways we send and receive messages. Handwriting and non-verbal aspects of communication, such as facial expression, body language and body posture, can also be affected.

In dealing with communication problems that arise, it can be helpful to think about how the different aspects of communication relate to each other as well as focusing on individual parts. Communication is about much more than speech, and the loss of communication skills in people with Parkinson's can create a misleading impression to those who come in contact with them.

We cannot stress too strongly the major contribution of effective communication to a good quality of life, and the importance, if you are experiencing difficulties, of obtaining early help and advice from a speech and language therapist You should either be able to refer yourself via your local hospital, or your doctor or Parkinson's Disease Nurse Specialist should be able to refer you.

Getting your message across

I look in the mirror and find it difficult to recognize myself, as my face seems so lacking in expression. Is there anything I can do to improve this?

Facial expression is a good example of an important kind of communication that is not speech. We all, perhaps without realizing, take a lot of notice of the facial expressions around us and it is often the first thing we notice about people. We may decide to give the boss a wide berth because he looks grumpy, or pass several people in the street before we see someone who looks friendly enough to ask for directions.

There are several things you can do to help yourself and the first is to try and maintain a good posture – there is a question about this in Chapter 9. If you can, try to look someone 'in the eye'. This will help with posture. Perhaps surprisingly, our second suggestion entails looking in the mirror! Facial exercises, for example frowning and screwing up your eyes, then moving down your face to grins, yawns and smiles, can help to keep the muscles of your face more mobile and are best done in front of a mirror. Try saying a suitable word or phrase while doing these exercises – you could say 'lovely to see you' when you smile, for example, or 'I'm bored to tears' when you yawn. So practise frowning, then opening and closing your eyes, wrinkling your nose, puffing out and sucking in your cheeks, whistling, smiling and yawning. A local speech and language therapist will be able to suggest other, individualized, exercises for you to try.

The third thing you can do is to tell your relations and friends that lack of facial expression is one of the symptoms of Parkinson's and that they should assume that your face may be giving out inaccurate messages. We are afraid that you may have to repeat this message many times because our normal response to facial expression is deeply ingrained and we can be disconcerted and upset by, for example, the absence of smiles, even when we have been told that it is a common symptom of Parkinson's. Partners, relatives and friends may need to be helped to understand and make allowances for this feature, especially in the early days after diagnosis. The PDS has information on all aspects of communication and Parkinson's. This includes tips for communicating with people with Parkinson's.

Are there particular exercises that I can do to help maintain my speech?

Yes there are, but which ones are most suitable will depend on how your speech is at the moment. A speech and language therapist can provide you with exercises and advice appropriate to your particular needs. Maintaining good posture and breathing is also important (see the previous question).

If you are already noticing some problems with your speech, you should contact your local Speech and Language Therapy Department as soon as possible (see Chapter 4 for more information about how to make contact with them). Do not be put off by mention of long waiting lists – ask at least to speak on the phone to a therapist with an interest in Parkinson's and explain your concerns. If talking on the phone is difficult, ask a family member or a friend to make the call for you.

I find that my voice is very quiet, almost a whisper. People – even my family – find it difficult to hear me. Can you suggest anything to help?

A weak or quiet voice is not uncommon and we would recommend that you seek an assessment from a speech and language therapist who will be able to suggest exercises tailored to your particular needs. Meanwhile, here are a few suggestions – you probably won't be able to follow them all the time, but keep trying and you will perhaps find things a little easier.

- Don't try to talk over noise, or from a different room.

- Try to keep your sentences short and precise.

- Think first what you want to say, then say it as simply as possible.

- Face the person you are talking to (people often lip read, which will help).

- Don't speak without taking a breath first.

- Enunciate (use your tongue, lips and jaw in a somewhat exaggerated way) very clearly. You may find this difficult, but try.

- You may find it helpful to imagine the room in which you are speaking is bigger than it really is.

- Your voice may tail off at the end of a sentence – try to make an extra effort here, or take a breath in during the sentence.

The problem of a quiet voice may be made worse if older family members have some loss of hearing. If this is suspected, do encourage them to seek help too.

I have many friends who live some distance away so I rely on the telephone. However, I find that the combined effect of my low voice and tremor are reducing my pleasure in these calls. Are there special phones which would help?

Yes. There are phones which you can use without holding the receiver, so helping to avoid problems from your tremor, and phones with amplifiers which will make your voice louder. Many phones now have memories, so you can store your most frequently used numbers and retrieve them by pushing just one or two buttons.

BT (British Telecom) has a special department to meet the needs of customers who have difficulties using the phone, and publishes a free guide called the *BT Guide for Disabled People* showing the equipment and services available. This can be obtained from their local sales offices, or you can telephone BT and they will send you a copy (see Appendix 2 for details). The Disabled Living Foundation has a useful fact sheet called *Choosing a Telephone, Textphone and Accessories* (see Appendix 2 for details).

My father's speech has become very hurried, so much so that the words run into each other and are sometimes incomprehensible. What could be done to help him slow down?

This is also a very common problem; it does sometimes happen and it is very frustrating for the person concerned and for their relatives and friends. Often this is linked to medication and to poor breath support. Try to get in touch with a speech and language therapist (see Chapter 4 for information about how to make contact), so that all aspects of your father's speech can be assessed. Encourage him to breathe deeply and steadily, to use short sentences and to vary the tone and volume of his voice as much as possible. The speech and language therapist will be able to suggest some exercises especially suited to his needs. Some people find tapping out a rhythm may help to slow them down.

The thing I find really frustrating about my Parkinson's is the way my whole way of behaving and speaking is inhibited and slowed down. Sometimes I am longing to add my comments to a conversation but I can't get started. Any suggestions?

You have drawn attention to some very important matters. We convey a lot about what we are and how we feel by the way we use our bodies. Actors make conscious use of this method of communication but the rest of us do it because we cannot help ourselves. It is called body language (for obvious reasons) and, as with loss of facial expression, relatives and friends can help to minimize the impact which it has on relationships and communication by being aware of what is happening. Ask them to read the information on communication produced by the PDS.

It would almost certainly be worth checking with your doctor to see if your Parkinson's medication could be changed in any way to improve your symptom control. Medication that improves your general condition may help your speech but will not necessarily do so. You should therefore contact a speech and language therapist at your local hospital or health centre for more detailed advice (see Chapter 4 for information on how to make contact with them).

Your relatives and friends also need to be discouraged from speaking for you or finishing your sentences for you, unless you have developed a deliberate strategy with someone to help you communicate. Even those of us who ought to know better sometimes break these important rules. Tell them you might use a signal like tapping or raising a hand to get in on the conversation.

Although he has had speech therapy in the past, my 55-year-old husband's speech is now quite poor and I think that we need an alternative method of communication. He is mentally alert but his hands are quite shaky so writing is not really possible. What choices do we have?

Your first and most important choice is to get in touch with your speech and language therapist again and see if she or he agrees with your assessment of the situation. If an alternative method of communication is needed, then the therapist will be able to help you consider which of a wide range of *communication aids* will best suit your husband's needs. These can range from alphabet boards and very individual sets of signals, to relatively small and simple machines such as Lightwriters to complex ones like computers. The most complex and expensive are not necessarily the best in every situation, so it is very important to discuss the situation with the speech and language therapist first. An advantage of the simpler systems such as cards or Lightwriters is that they are portable and so can be taken into less familiar situations, for example day centres or hospitals, where communication problems can be especially distressing. An advantage of the more complex (and expensive) systems, like computers, is that they may open up new interests for your husband, if he has the patience and the will to learn how to use them. You will find more about this in the section on *Leisure* in the next chapter.

8
Work and leisure

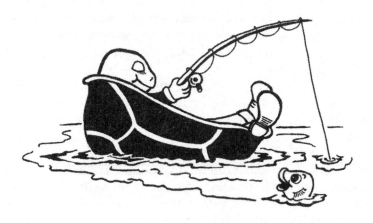

For people still in full-time work, the onset of a permanent condition like Parkinson's can create considerable anxieties and uncertainties. In a climate of economic recession, such anxieties are exacerbated. Those who have decided to give up work or who have already retired face similar concerns about their capacity to go on doing the things that they enjoy – the things reflecting their personalities and helping to make life worthwhile. The questions in this chapter are about these very important aspects of life and, like the questions in all the other chapters, they underline the great diversity of people with Parkinson's and the need to find individual solutions.

Work

I am 44 and was diagnosed 18 months ago. I am an estate agent. For how long can I expect to continue working?

This sort of question is always difficult to answer because Parkinson's varies so much from one person to another. As you don't say how well you are at the moment, it is especially difficult to give you a clear answer. With effective medication, people with Parkinson's can often continue working for many years. The introduction of apomorphine (which acts very quickly) means that, in people whom it suits, there is now even more chance of staying in employment. (See Chapter 3 for more information about apomorphine.)

It is easier to carry on working in some kinds of employment than others, especially in those that do not require great physical stamina or fast reaction times. Sometimes people with Parkinson's take early retirement, not because they cannot manage the job, but because they eventually find that the stress of work is interfering with their overall quality of life. The point at which a reduction in stress and more time for other activities outweighs the various advantages of remaining at work will be different for each person. Your eligibility for benefits and overall financial situation will, of course, be an important consideration, and you may find it helpful to read the rest of this section and parts of Chapter 12.

I work as a teacher in a large inner city school. It's interesting and challenging work but also stressful. Should I consider early retirement?

There is no 'should' involved here. Everything depends on how you feel, what your quality of life is while at work and whether, in order to keep working, you have to give up lots of the other activities which make life worthwhile.

Retiring from work is one of life's major turning points and should not be rushed into without balancing all the pros and cons. In this sense, you should certainly consider carefully before making such an important decision. Do not make a big decision like this if you are currently feeling depressed or shocked, for example because you have just been given the diagnosis. You should also be sure to give any new Parkinson's treatment adequate time to have an effect before making such decisions.

The financial implications of early retirement are often an important part of the equation (there is a question about this in Chapter 12), and it is vital that you obtain some good advice from a competent person. Often a personnel officer, a professional association or trade union is able to offer such advice, but, if not, you could approach the Welfare and Employment Rights Department at the Parkinson's Disease Society (address in Appendix 1). Their employment pack includes information on retiring early on medical grounds.

Should I tell the people at work that I have Parkinson's? The treatment is working well but I know that there are some tell-tale signs and that I am slower than I used to be.

There is no answer to this question which is right for everyone, although we believe that the balance of advantage usually lies in telling the most important people such as your closest colleague and your immediate manager. If you are aware of 'tell-tale signs', the chances are that your colleagues at work have seen them too and are drawing their own conclusions. Their interpretations may be quite wrong and less complimentary than the truth! As we mentioned in Chapter 2, stress can make the symptoms of Parkinson's worse and, once you stop having to cover up, you may actually be able to do your job better.

However, there will be circumstances, especially in a recession, when all jobs are at risk. Only you can know whether this risk is sufficiently grave in your own work situation to outweigh these arguments. We discuss these issues further in the answer to the next question.

What effects might my diagnosis have on my job security?

As we suggested at the end of the previous answer, much depends on the kind of work you do and the general level of job security in your firm or employment sector. Obviously any kind of long-term illness can have an effect on job security. If your Parkinson's seems likely to have an early impact on your ability to do your present job, you should discuss this with your doctor to see if the treatment could be improved in any way. When you understand the medical situation fully, you should sit down and discuss the situation with someone who will help you to think through your options. You will find suggestions about whom this 'someone' might be in the answer to the next question. There is also a question further on in this chapter about how to obtain information on alternative jobs and retraining, and questions in Chapter 12 about the financial aspects.

What is important to note is that the Disability Discrimination Act 1995 now protects people with disabilities in a number of areas including employment. The Act covers discrimination against people who either have a disability or have had a disability in the past. Disability is defined as a physical or mental impairment, which has a substantial and long-term effect on a person's ability to carry out normal day-to-day activities. Since the end of 1998 it has been unlawful for an employer with 15 or more employees to discriminate against disabled people in a number of situations, (the number is changing from October 2004). Unless the treatment can be justified, it would be unlawful for an employer to treat a person less favourably for a reason related to their disability. It would also be unlawful for an employer to refuse to make a 'reasonable adjustment' within the work place to enable a disabled person to work. There will be further changes to the Disability Discrimination Act in October 2004. The PDS Welfare and Employment Rights Department, Disability Rights Commission or the Disability Services Team at your local Jobcentre Plus office can advise further. The PDS also has information sheets on *Employment* (WB11) and *The Disability Discrimination Act* (FS53).

What action should I take if I have problems in coping with my work or if my employer is not very understanding?

There are really two questions here. The first is about coping with work. It would be helpful to begin by clarifying in your own mind what the problems are. Then you need to talk things over with a good listener, preferably someone who knows about Parkinson's. You may know someone suitable already but, if not, you could contact the Parkinson's Disease Society and talk to either the Welfare and Employment Rights Department or the Helpline staff. There may also be a PDS community support worker in your area with whom you could discuss things. They will be able to help you identify other sources of advice and information which might include your doctor, your employer and employment disability services.

The second question relates to what you should do if your employer is not very understanding. The first actions would be those just described but you would need to add some consideration of the ways in which he or she is unhelpful, and the chances of change if the situation was properly explained. Try talking to your boss and see if your workload can be adjusted, or get an advocate to talk to your employer for you. The variable symptoms of Parkinson's can cause misunderstandings if the person concerned has not come across it before. If your conclusion is that your employer's attitude cannot be improved, then the balance would tip in favour of trying to find alternative employment or considering early retirement. The organizations mentioned in the previous question should also be able to advise. See also the information about the Disability Discrimination Act 1995 in the previous question.

My husband is a qualified accountant but is unable to drive so is off work. Is there any way he could be helped to work from home?

Working from home is no longer uncommon – indeed, some people suggest that it is where nearly everyone will be working in the fairly near future. It can be particularly feasible for professional people who do not require lots of expensive equipment. Home computers that can be linked to those in the office offer many new possibilities of work from home. Your husband should first talk to his current firm to explore what options they can offer.

If they cannot offer home work, he could approach the Placing, Assessment and Counselling Team (PACT) at his local Jobcentre Plus (listed under 'Employment Service' in the phone book or see the Jobcentre Plus website listed in Appendix 1). PACT has disability employment advisers who can offer a range of services to people with disabilities. It can help to be registered with the Employment Service as disabled and this can be arranged through these advisers. We understand that accepting the label 'disabled' can be a difficult step to take but, if your husband can get over this hurdle, he will gain access to many sources of help. To qualify for registration you have to be 'a person who, on account of injury, disease or congenital deformity, is substantially handicapped in obtaining or keeping employment, or in undertaking work on his own account of a kind which would be suited to his age, experience and qualification'. The disability must be likely to last at least 12 months and the person concerned must be either in, or actively looking for, work and have some prospect of getting it. Among the services available to people so registered are free permanent loans of equipment, which helps to obtain or keep employment and help with fares to work where driving is inappropriate.

If your husband is thinking of working independently from home, it will be worth doing some research into the possibilities and pitfalls. Any unemployed person can apply for help to set up a small business through the Business Start-up Scheme run by the Training and Enterprise Councils (TECs) or in Scotland by the Local Enterprise Companies (LECs). Any Jobcentre Plus will have more details. There is also an association called the Telecottage Association (see Appendix 1 for their telephone number), which provides information and a support network for people working from home.

The other issue raised by your question is whether you have explored all the options for helping him to get to work. You will find more about this in Chapter 11 on *Getting around on wheels*.

Is specialized advice available about possible alternative jobs and retraining?

Yes. As mentioned in the previous answer, your local Jobcentre Plus has a disability employment adviser who has special responsibility for helping people with a disability to find appropriate work. This includes retraining if necessary and any government schemes that may be appropriate for someone with Parkinson's. Employment policy is in a state of constant flux and the criteria for admission to the various training schemes are detailed and complex, so it is best to discuss your personal requirements with the adviser.

There are also private careers consultants who offer individualized advice although, of course, there is a charge for their services. To locate them, look in your local Yellow Pages under Careers Advice or Personnel Consultants.

Alternatively you could approach the Welfare and Employment Rights Department at the Parkinson's Disease Society (details in Chapter 15 and address in Appendix 1).

Leisure

My Parkinson's came on very slowly and has only recently been recognized. Meanwhile I seem to have given up lots of my old interests. Should I try to pick them up again now I'm receiving treatment?

Yes, definitely. We cannot emphasize too strongly the importance of keeping active and living as normal a life as possible. Your experience is not unusual when the symptoms come on very gradually, and it is a good sign that you are now thinking of picking up some of your old interests. Try one or two for a start, especially those you enjoyed most or which kept you in touch with friends, and see how things go.

My husband has always been interested in sport – as a player rather than a watcher. Are there any sports which seem particularly suitable for people with Parkinson's?

We know of people with Parkinson's who play almost every kind of sport, so there is sure to be something suitable for your husband. Energetic team games may pose some problems but tennis, squash, badminton, bowls, swimming, walking and snooker are just a few among many other possibilities. There are special organizations promoting sport for people with disabilities in the four countries within the United Kingdom (see the various sports addresses in Appendix 1) whom he could contact if he has difficulty finding suitable local facilities, although many sports centres now make special provision for people with disabilities.

The PDS has published a booklet called *At Your Leisure* (B75) which provides information on sport and leisure activities which are suitable for people with Parkinson's.

One friend has told me that I will have to give up the active things I enjoy doing (which are dancing, walking, cycling and gardening) now that I have Parkinson's. Another friend disagreed, and said that it would be much better for me to keep on with them. Who's right?

There is no need for you to give up your activities because of your Parkinson's. Almost any form of exercise that you enjoy and that you can carry on safely and without undue fatigue is beneficial. The benefit comes in lots of different ways: physically in keeping your body fit and your joints and muscles in good condition; emotionally through the enjoyment and the sense of achievement; and socially because you get out to meet people and have things to think or talk about other than your Parkinson's. If you have any doubts about your chosen form of exercise, check with your doctor first.

The special advantages of music therapy are discussed in Chapter 3. Gardening is dealt with in the next question. The PDS publication *At Your Leisure* (B75) also has information on all these activities.

Gardening has been one of the passions in my life but the physical effort involved is beginning to detract from my enjoyment. Is there some way I can make things easier?

We sympathize – gardening is a major source of exercise, fresh air, creativity and enjoyment for millions of people and it is important to retain this interest for as long as possible. Luckily you are not the first person to feel this way and there are two organizations which provide advice and practical help to gardeners with disabilities, Gardening for the Disabled Trust and Thrive (see Appendix 1 for the addresses).

Other general information sources such as DIAL (Disablement Information Advice Lines) and the Disabled Living Foundation are also likely to have information about aids and equipment for gardeners. There is also an invaluable paperback full of good advice and information about equipment, seeds, manufacturers and relevant organizations. Called *Grow It Yourself* (details in Appendix 2), it will answer many of your questions and encourage you to continue cultivating your passion!

My wife, who has Parkinson's, and I have moved around the country a lot and have many old friends we would like to visit. However, I am also somewhat disabled with arthritis and cannot drive any more. Is there anywhere we could get help in planning journeys to accommodate our combined disabilities?

Yes. There is an organization called Tripscope (details in Appendix 1) which specializes in helping to plan travel for people with disabilities. If you are travelling by rail, look under 'Railways' in your local phone book and telephone any organization that offers help to people with disabilities. They should be able to arrange any necessary help throughout the journey, as well as booking your tickets. If you need an escort, you can usually get assistance from St John Ambulance or the British Red Cross and sometimes from local service organizations such as Rotary, Round Table, Lions or Soroptimists. Your local Citizens Advice should be able to give you details of local groups. See also the PDS Welfare and Employment Rights Department's information sheet, *Help with Getting Around* (W10).

Would it be unwise to try to travel by air to Canada on my own? I am still active but carrying cases would be a strain.

Many people with Parkinson's enjoy international travel and there is no obvious reason why you should not go to Canada on your own. It will be sensible to choose a schedule which is not too demanding and which allows you to rest after the journey. If your only health problem is Parkinson's and the only foreseeable problem is coping with the luggage, then travelling by air is one of the safest and easiest means of travel. Airlines are particularly good about looking after passengers who need extra help, especially if you notify them beforehand. Check with your doctor anyway, just in case he or she has any special advice to offer.

Make sure that you take a good supply of your medicines and also a doctor's letter stating clearly what has been prescribed. This will be useful for your hosts if, by chance, you are unwell or need extra supplies, and will help avoid any possible problems at customs, etc. It is a good idea to have supplies of medicine in two separate bags so that, if one goes missing, you still have a supply.

Publications you might find helpful include the PDS information sheet, *International Travel* (FS28), the Disabled Living Foundation's book, *Flying High,* and the Department of Health leaflet, *Traveller's Guide to Health* (see Appendix 2 for how to obtain copies). You should also ensure that you have adequate holiday insurance and that you have given full information to your insurers about your Parkinson's and any other permanent medical condition. It is worth comparing quotes for insurance before choosing your policy, as the costs can vary considerably, but be sure to read the small print so that you know what level of cover is on offer. Bon voyage!

My husband has always enjoyed writing – letters, diaries, poems, etc. – and is very frustrated by how bad his handwriting has become. What can you suggest to help him maintain his interest in writing?

Deteriorating handwriting is a great source of frustration to many people with Parkinson's even if they do not also share your husband's literary interests. Simple solutions to handwriting problems include a thick or padded pen or pencil, which can help improve grip and control. Weighted pens or wrist bands help some people and Dycem mats (which are made of washable, slightly sticky plastic) can stop the paper from sliding around. Your local occupational therapist (see Chapter 4 for how to make contact) will be able to offer advice on all these options and is also likely to have some suggestions about how the legibility of handwriting can be improved. See the PDS information sheet *Handwriting* (FS23) for more information.

Another option is a personal computer, word processor or electronic typewriter. The keyboards require less effort than old-fashioned manual typewriters, and computers or word processors allow the written material to be corrected, amended and re-arranged any number of times before it is printed. There is software available that will adjust for the tremor in Parkinson's.

Try to get some good advice before you buy as there are so many competing models and packages on the market. We would suggest you contact AbilityNet (see Appendix 1 for the address), an organization which provides advice on computers and IT to people with disabilities. We know of several people with Parkinson's whose lives have been transformed by access to a personal computer. (Please see Chapter 12 on *Finance* for information about obtaining help with the cost of computers.) See the PDS information sheet, *Computers and the Internet* (FS60).

If a computer is the chosen solution and your husband needs training in how to use it, then local further education colleges or adult education facilities should have a range of courses in computing. We even know of people with Parkinson's who have been provided with home tutors. He may also be able to do a course through LearnDirect, a government sponsored initiative in flexible learning involving a network on online learning and information services. AbilityNet may also be able to advise on training. (See Appendix 1 for contact details.)

One last suggestion – your husband may want to extend his interest in writing by joining a writers' group or class. There are many different kinds of opportunities, ranging from local further education courses to residential courses lasting for a weekend or even longer. The PDS publication *At Your Leisure* (B75) also has a section on continuing education and development.

Reading has been a source of pleasure throughout my life but is now becoming quite difficult owing to a combination of Parkinson's tremor and failing eyesight. Are there any aids or organizations which might help?

In answering this question we assume that you have sought medical advice about both the tremor and your eyesight. When you are on the best possible treatment, there are several other things you can do to help preserve this invaluable hobby. You will find details of all the organizations mentioned below in Appendix 1.

An occupational therapist could advise you on ways of making holding a book easier. There are book stands which will help to hold the book steady (ask your occupational therapist or contact the Disabled Living Foundation, a local Disabled Living Centre or one of the shops to see what is available). There are also large print books (Ulverscroft and Chivers are two of the largest publishers) and books on cassette available in bookshops and in most public libraries. Talking books are also available from Listening Books (this service is available to all people with disabilities, not just those with impaired vision). There are also some newspapers on cassette available from the Talking Newspapers Association UK. Lastly, if there are particular papers, books or documents which you wish to read, large public libraries often have special machines which can magnify text or turn it into spoken words. You usually have to make a booking for these machines. (See Appendix 1 for contact details.)

We love going to the theatre and concerts but my husband's Parkinson's, which causes quite a lot of tremor and involuntary movements, is beginning to make this difficult. Do you have any ideas to help?

Our advice would be to contact the management of any cinema, theatre or concert hall you want to attend and explain the situation. Managements have begun to be much more aware of the requirements of people with special needs but, to date, they seem to have mainly considered the needs of people in wheelchairs and those with hearing difficulties.

For your particular problem, there may be some seats which would be especially suitable, or you may find that matinée performances are less crowded and so less likely to cause problems of distraction to others and embarrassment to your husband.

London has an information service called Artsline, which provides information on arts events for people with disabilities. It would be worth checking with your nearest DIAL (Disablement Information Advice Lines – contact DIAL UK at the address in Appendix 1 for details of your local DIAL) or local authority information service whether there is anything similar in your area.

If you feel that you would like to campaign for improved access to public places for people with disabilities, you may find that you have a local Access group doing just that.

The Disability Discrimination Act 1995, mentioned earlier in this chapter in the employment section, also covers access to goods, services and facilities including theatres. See the PDS information sheet on the *Disability Discrimination Act* (FS53) for more details.

I am a crossword and board game fanatic but am finding it increasingly difficult to cope with the fine hand movements required. How can I keep up my interest?

The various sources of aids mentioned in previous answers in this chapter, particularly the Disabled Living Foundation and the Disabled Living Centres, will have some games which are easier to manage. However, the best source of such games is now the home computer for which you can obtain crosswords, chess, bridge and many other traditional games as well as a vast array of modern computer games. There are many computer magazines on sale and in libraries which will have articles and advertisements about games programs. AbilityNet, the organization already mentioned, advises disabled people on computers and they might be able to provide information on what is available. They can also advise on any adaptations you might need to overcome any problems with fine hand movements that might restrict your use of a computer and computer games.

Now that I have retired, I would like to fill some of the gaps in my formal education and general knowledge. What options do I have?

A huge number. Apart from colleges of further and higher education which are making special efforts to make their courses accessible to non-traditional students, there is also the Open University, Open College of the Arts and the University of the Third Age (see Appendix 1 for addresses). All these organizations offer a wide range of courses and methods of learning, and cover academic subjects, current affairs, art, music, languages and much, much more.

My husband and I love visiting stately homes, old houses, gardens and so on, but sometimes they turn out to be unsuitable for his wheelchair and we end up being very disappointed. Is there some way of finding out whether a place is suitable in advance?

You can, of course, telephone most places in advance and it is certainly worth doing this if you are planning to travel a considerable distance. For general planning of outings and to cut down on telephone calls there are several useful publications.

For example, the *National Trust Handbook* gives information about the suitability of its properties for people in wheelchairs, has a specific leaflet for visitors with disabilities, which can also be downloaded from their website. Some National Trust properties have motorized buggies available for people with mobility problems, and all give free admission to someone escorting a disabled person. Other books giving details of wheelchair access are the *National Gardens Scheme Handbook*, and *Historic Houses, Castles and Gardens* which includes 'over 1300 historic properties from cottages to castles'. Details of all these publications are in Appendix 2.

Other sources of information are RADAR (the Royal Association for Disability and Rehabilitation – their address is in Appendix 1) or, for ideas about places quite near to your home, try contacting some of the local groups for people with disabilities.

9
Managing at home

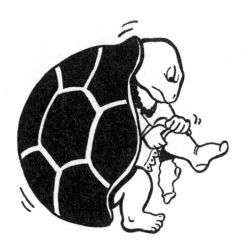

With appropriate medication, adequate exercise and a healthy lifestyle, many people with Parkinson's have few difficulties in managing everyday tasks around the home. However, from the beginning quite a few have other medical conditions as well as Parkinson's, and so may meet additional problems. Others find that, as the years pass, things that were easy become more troublesome. Remember that it is unlikely that anyone will have all the difficulties mentioned in this chapter so you need to find the questions that apply to you or to your partner, family member or friend.

There is a balance for everyone between independence and the selective use of equipment or new ways of approaching tasks – you may need to experiment to find out what is right for you. Although it can sometimes be hard to accept the need to make changes, a new tool or technique can mean a real extension of independence for many people.

Mobility and safety

Getting up out of a chair is a real problem – do you have any advice that will help?

Our first advice is to make sure that your regular chair is the right height for you, i.e. not too low, that it is stable and has arms from which you can push up as you rise. Sometimes you may be able to adapt your present chair or you may want to buy a new one. You can either get advice from a reputable mobility shop that stocks equipment for people with mobility problems, and whose staff are trained to look at your needs, or from professionals such as physiotherapists, occupational therapists or appropriate social services department staff. Once you are sure that your chair is suitable, try the following sequence of actions.

1. Move to the edge of the chair.
2. Place your feet flat on the floor, well under you.
3. Position your feet 8–10 inches apart.
4. Put your hands on the arms of the chair (or on the sides of the chair seat).
5. Now lean forwards as far as you can from your hips. This is very important to allow your bottom to rise up off the chair seat.
6. Push up through your arms and keep your body moving forwards and upwards (your nose should be in line with your toes).
7. Keep pushing until you are standing up. When you have your balance in this upright position, it is safe to let go of the chair arms.

I sometimes get stuck when approaching a doorway or narrow passage. Why should this happen and what can I do to solve the problem?

What you describe is a form of 'freezing', when you get stuck and cannot seem to get going again. It is thought that freezing occurs when a normal sequence of movement is interrupted, although its exact cause is not clearly understood. Freezing becomes noticeably worse if a person is anxious, in an unfamiliar situation or loses concentration. It can occur in a number of places or situations but particularly when approaching a doorway or elevator, when passing through narrow spaces, in crowded or new places and when the surface a person is walking on changes suddenly, such as a different pattern on a carpet or a change from a smooth to an uneven surface.

Freezing is one of the aspects of Parkinson's in which a whole range of 'try it yourself' solutions have grown up, as many people with Parkinson's have developed their own ways of getting themselves moving. All these solutions emphasize putting your heels to the ground first, to help you regain your balance and to keep it as you move. Once your heels are down, you can 'choose' from a whole range of options, including rocking from side to side, swivelling your head and shoulders to look at something alongside you, marching on the spot, swinging your leg backwards before trying to move forwards, stepping over imaginary lines, or even thinking 'provocative thoughts'! See the PDS information sheet, *Freezing* (FS63) for more information.

How important is good posture and what can I do to maintain it?

Good posture is very important and can have an influence on many of the other things you want to do, such as walking, balancing and talking. There seems to be a natural tendency for people to become a bit stooped or round-shouldered as they get older and this tendency is exaggerated with Parkinson's.

You may be surprised to learn that posture can affect talking, but this is because stooping constricts the lungs and makes it more difficult to breathe properly. So improving your posture can help prevent or alleviate speech difficulties (see Chapter 7 for more about speech and communication).

The first step towards improving your posture is to be aware of it. You can do this by standing or sitting in front of a mirror, noting your posture and trying to correct any faults you see. Study your 'improved' posture and then allow yourself to relax back into your normal posture. You should be able to feel as well as see the difference.

Here are a couple of exercises which will help you improve your posture and 'stand tall'. For the first, stand with your back against a wall and with the backs of your heels touching it. Now try to stand up as straight as you can so that your shoulder blades and the back of your head also touch the wall (see Figure 9.1, left). Try and hold the position at least for a slow count of five, and then relax. Repeat this a few times.

For the second exercise, you should stand facing the wall and a few inches away from it. Put the palms of your hands against

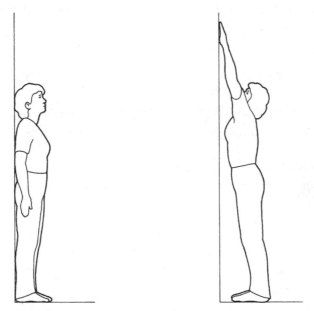

Figure 9.1 Posture exercises

the wall and stretch up as high as you can, watching your hands all the time (see Figure 9.1, right). When you have stretched up as far as you can, hold the position for at least a slow count of five, and then relax. Again, repeat this exercise a few times.

Encourage your closest relative or friend to remind you to keep a good posture and it should get easier, though perhaps never easy.

What are the rules for turning round safely?

Never swivel on one foot or cross your legs. Walk round in a semicircle, with your feet slightly apart. In other words, make the turn part of your walk. Always turn in a forward direction.

We would add the following rules, especially for situations where there is a shortage of space.

1. Get your balance first before you start to turn.

2. Take your time – don't rush.

3. Do it in stages, for example make four quarter turns rather than one big one.

How can I improve my walking? I have a tendency to take very short steps or to shuffle.

Parkinson's can affect walking in lots of different ways and the effect varies from person to person and from one time to another. It's important to try to find the solution that is right for you because walking is an excellent form of exercise as well as a way of maintaining your independence and keeping up your interests and activities. Some of the following suggestions may help.

- Stop and take stock if you feel things are going wrong.

- Stand as straight as possible – leaning forward makes it more likely that you will either go too fast or get stuck.

- When you step forward, put your heel down first as your foot comes into contact with the ground, and then your toe.

- Give yourself spoken instructions such as 'heel, heel' as you go along. People with Parkinson's find that sometimes such a cue or prompt, either from themselves, or someone else or using a rhythm such as a musical or metronome beat, can help improve stepping.

These suggestions are things which you can do for yourself, but there are physiotherapists with special experience in Parkinson's who could give you expert, individualized advice. To obtain this, you should ask your doctor to refer you to a physiotherapist (see Chapter 4 for information about making contact).

I've always hated the idea of walking with a stick but now feel rather unsteady and am tempted to stay indoors. What walking aids are available?

We will assume that you have consulted your doctor and a physiotherapist so that your walking has been improved as much as possible. An ordinary walking stick with a non-slip ferrule (a rubber tip) does give some people quite a bit more confidence so we think you should probably try that first. Perhaps you could consider having an interesting or unusual stick or even a selection of different ones for different occasions! There are even trendy ferrules for trekking poles. There are other walking aids such as tripod sticks, walking frames with and without wheels, folding frames, and trolleys but they are more for use inside the house than outside. However, if you are unfamiliar with their use, they can actually be a hazard and put you at risk of tripping over them. Make sure you get advice from a physiotherapist or occupational therapist before you buy, or buy from a reputable supplier that has staff who can advise and where they will let you have one on trial. Walking-length umbrellas are **not** a good idea, as they are not secure enough to lean on.

If you do find you need anything more than a walking stick, it is really important to be properly assessed by a physiotherapist who understands about Parkinson's, as not all walking aids are suitable for people with Parkinson's.

Getting out and keeping up your interests is important so it is good that you are willing to revise your attitude towards something that may help. Confidence can also be boosted by having someone to accompany you when you go out. You may even want to consider 'wheels' some time, in which case you could look at the questions and answers in Chapter 11.

My wife gets really frustrated by her inability to turn over in bed and it's causing her to have bad nights. Can you suggest anything to help?

This is a little understood but very common symptom of Parkinson's – in one survey of members of the PDS, more than 60% reported this problem. Although there is unlikely to be a complete solution for her problem, there are several things which can help. We assume that your wife has checked her current medication with her doctor to ensure that it is at its best.

Having checked the medication, next check the bed! It is often easier to turn over on a firm mattress (if it is too soft, you could try putting a board underneath it). An occupational therapist can advise on the bed and may also be able to suggest other ways of making turning over in bed easier. Some people find silk or satin sheets useful, as they allow easier movement, or your wife could try wearing silk or satin nightwear. Bedsocks may also make it easier to get a grip and so help turning over. You might also find the PDS information sheet, *Sleep and Night-time Problems* (FS30) helpful.

I live alone and getting out of bed (I have to, several times a night) is really difficult. Is there an aid which would help?

We do not have enough information to consider whether your need to get out of bed so often could be tackled. However, we would suggest you consider why you need to get out of bed so often. Is it because you need to go to the toilet, or because you are restless and having trouble sleeping? Some other reason? It might be a good idea to discuss this with your doctor, as there might be solutions that would reduce the number of times you have to get out of bed in the night.

With regard to help to get yourself out of bed, this depends on the exact nature of your difficulty. Rather than a piece of equipment, the answer may be to learn some techniques for getting yourself, by easy stages, into the right position. The person to advise you further is an occupational therapist. They could also advise on any small pieces of equipment that might be helpful, such as a bed pull which lies on top of the covers or a special frame by the side of the bed. If your main difficulty is getting into a sitting position, you could consider an electrically operated bed, mattress or part-mattress. However, it is important to seek advice from the occupational therapist before buying anything to ensure what you buy is appropriate for your needs. See also the PDS information sheet *Sleep and Night-time Problems* (FS30) and *Living Alone* (FS29).

How can I reduce the risks of falling in the house?

In two ways. Firstly you can organize your home so that it is free from potential hazards such as slippery, polished floors, loose rugs and mats, trailing electric cables, and general clutter left on the floor. It will also help if you arrange your furniture to make moving around the house as easy as possible (for example, make sure that you don't have to avoid the coffee table every time you walk from your sitting room to the kitchen to get a cup of tea). Keep an eye open for pets – an affectionate cat or overenthusiastic dog could also create hazards.

Secondly, you need to make sure that you are walking, turning round and getting out of your chair and so on as safely as possible (we have covered these topics in answers to earlier questions in this chapter). A special word of warning against reaching out for furniture to support yourself when moving around the house. Doing this could make falls more likely. See the PDS information sheet, *Falls* (FS39) for more information. An occupational therapist could also advise further.

Although it is easy for us to say 'don't rush', we know that it is difficult to break the habits of a lifetime. However, **do try not to** and, if there are particular occasions which tempt you to rush, such as the telephone ringing, consider placing a phone next to your usual chair, having some extra phones installed or switching to a cordless phone. See also the question on telephones in Chapter 7 on *Communication*.

I have always enjoyed being a housewife and making my home attractive. Now people keep telling me to make it safe and I'm afraid it won't look like a home any more – and then I'll lose interest.

There is an important balancing act to be done here and we sympathize with your feelings about wanting to keep your home feeling like home. However, with good advice from an occupational therapist and a little imagination and ingenuity from you, it ought to be possible to achieve something which is both reasonably safe and homelike.

We have to acknowledge that there can be no perfectly safe environment – and, if there were, its inhabitants would probably die of boredom! – so it's a question of compromise. It is also true that caring relatives and friends can become overprotective. You may need to sit down with them and talk about the freedoms you need and want to retain, and to acknowledge that the situation can be difficult for everyone involved.

I like to do my own cooking and cleaning but get tired easily and some days find such activities quite impossible. Do you have any tips which might help?

The first and most important tip is to time such chores for when you are at your best and to be prepared (with convenience foods and a conveniently blind eye for dust, etc.) for days when you need more rest.

Of course we all use many labour-saving devices for preparing food and cleaning nowadays and you should make the maximum use of these. Items such as food processors can make a big difference. The kitchen especially needs to be organized in such a way that it is as safe and energy-efficient as possible. The expert in this field is the occupational therapist and, if you have not already requested a visit through either your GP or social services department, you should do so as soon as possible (see Chapter 4 for more information about making contact). If appropriate, she or he will also be able to recommend equipment especially suited to your needs. Some items are very simple, such as non-slip mats to hold mixing bowls, padded handles, high stools and trolleys. Others are more expensive and he or she may suggest a visit to your nearest Disabled Living Centre to try various models before deciding what to buy (see Appendix 1 for the Disabled Living Centres Council's address – they will give you details of your nearest centre).

Cooking can be a rewarding and enjoyable hobby as well as a practical necessity, so it is a good idea to try to maintain this interest.

Personal care

I pride myself on keeping clean and fresh but it's not easy with stiff limbs and a tremor. There must be others, men and women, in the same boat. How can we find out what items of equipment are available?

There are many items of equipment available to help with personal care. These range from simple things like long-handled sponges to expensive specialized items like lavatories that can wash and dry. The Disabled Living Foundation publish information sheets on all kinds of equipment and have centres where you can try out equipment and get advice from a therapist. The Disabled Living Centres Council can advise you where your nearest one is. Commercial companies such as Keep Able also sell many of these items and offer mail order/online shopping.

However, if you need anything other than very simple items, we suggest that you get advice from an occupational therapist first. Sometimes it is not just a question of the right piece of equipment but of how you tackle the task in question. An occupational therapist will be able to advise further.

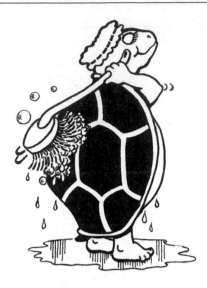

My mother, aged 75, loves to have a 'proper' bath but slipped recently in the bath and has lost confidence. I realize that we could have a shower fitted but is there any other solution to her problem?

One of the authors was once told that showers were all right for getting clean but if you wanted a deep, emotional experience, then a 'proper' bath was necessary! We think it is easy for professionals to underestimate the importance of baths as relaxation, especially for older people, so your question is an important one.

There are several lines of approach. You could try to help your mother feel more confident again by getting her to practise (with bare feet, of course, to prevent slipping) getting in and out of the bath while you are present. It can also help enormously if you, or someone else with whom she feels comfortable, can be around when she has a bath. There is also a wide range of appliances such as rails, mats and bath seats that might help, An occupational therapist could advise further. See Chapter 4 for details of how to make contact.

You could request help with bathing by asking for a community care assessment. See Chapter 4 for more information about these. Who provides bathing services depends on your local area.

In some places it will be social services and in others the Primary Care Trust. There is a question on bathing services in Chapter 4.

Another possibility is to see if there is a local nursing home which offers day care. Some of them have a variety of baths including 'walk-in' models, one of which might be especially suitable for your mother. Nearly all of these solutions might cost something depending on the arrangements in your local area and your mother's income. Using the nursing home would almost certainly be the most expensive unless the social services department agreed to provide it as part of a community care package (see Chapter 4 for more details).

I have been told that good dental hygiene is important and I do try, but manipulating a toothbrush is now quite difficult. Is there anything which would help?

You are right about good dental hygiene being important – a healthy mouth and strong teeth contribute to good appearance and good diet. A padded handle on your toothbrush might help and some people find an electric toothbrush very useful. As with any other activities which you find difficult or tiring, you should choose a time of the day when your medication is working reasonably well. Mouthwashes, or chewing gum between brushing, may also be helpful. Be sure to keep in regular touch with your dentist (see Chapter 4 if finding a suitable one causes any difficulties).

It is also worth noting that any tasks such as brushing teeth, shaving, drying hair, and so on (all of which require controlled hand and arm movements) may be easier and less tiring if you support your elbows on a dressing table or other flat surface. Your dentist or an occupational therapist might be able to advise further. See also the booklet *Parkinson's and Dental Health* (B45).

The monthly discomfort of my period is made worse by the practical problems of my Parkinson's. What advice can you offer?

This is a difficult question to answer because the information on how Parkinson's affects younger women is limited. However, in recent years the PDS Helpline has received quite a lot of anecdotal information from young women regarding gynaecological problems and their monthly cycle. There has been a study in the USA in which 75% of the women noted worsening of their symptoms before and during their period.

First you need to talk with your doctor to ensure that both your Parkinson's and your periods are being managed as well as they can be. Some neurologists, working with a gynaecologist colleague, may alter the dosage of levodopa during menstruation.

If you can arrange your social diary to avoid very strenuous activity during this time it might avoid further frustration because, although you do not want Parkinson's and menstruation to rule your life, you do want to enjoy any special events to the full. If you have Parkinson's Disease Nurse Specialist, they might be able to advise you.

You can feel very isolated with this kind of problem because the number of younger women with Parkinson's is relatively small, so you may like to consider joining the YAPP&RS (see Chapter 15 for more information). This is a special section of the Parkinson's Disease Society for younger people, which enables you to exchange ideas with people who are likely to share some of your problems.

I have some gynaecological problems and I need to talk to someone about what can be done and how allowance can be made for the effects of my Parkinson's – I have both 'off' times and fairly severe involuntary movements. Who could help me think things through?

As we said in the previous answer, the number of younger women with Parkinson's is relatively small so there are hardly any people around with the sort of combined expertise that you need. There is some interest amongst Parkinson's specialists in the effects of hormones on Parkinson's and daily living skills but little documentation. One of the first things to do would be talk to your Parkinson's consultant who might be able to suggest some strategies for dealing with your particular problems or have a gynaecologist colleague with whom he or she could work with to try and resolve your problems. Other sources of possible help might be a Parkinson's Disease Nurse Specialist, one of the nurses on the PDS Helpline or other women with Parkinson's who are members of YAPP&Rs, the PDS's special interest group for younger people with Parkinson's, and who are experiencing similar problems.

You do not state what your gynaecological problems are and whether they will necessitate surgery. Generally speaking people with Parkinson's can undergo general surgery but again, because gynaecological problems involve female hormones, and because these have an effect on people's Parkinson's, it requires careful management. It might be helpful if you kept a diary for the next month or two so that you have some pattern regarding your problems when you next see either consultant.

Dressing and undressing is such a hassle for people with Parkinson's especially if they live alone like me. What sorts of clothes are best and where can I find a good selection?

Yes, dressing and undressing can be difficult, and suitable clothes can make an important contribution to easing the problem. However, it is also important to choose a time when your tablets are working reasonably well and a place where you can be comfortable so that you can take your time. An occupational therapist should be able to advise further on aspects of dressing and clothes that might make it easier for you to manage.

Today's casual clothes with their elasticated waistbands and baggy tops can be ideal for people with dressing problems, and have the added advantage that you can look like everyone else if you wish. Velcro, which is now used for fastenings on everything from waistbands to shoes, has been a great boon to people who have difficulty getting dressed.

The Parkinson's Disease Society publishes an information sheet on *Clothing* (FS31) and there are also some special mail-order catalogue selections of clothes for people with dressing problems, including J D Williams & Company Ltd. The Disabled Living Foundation has several information sheets on dressing and a book called *All Dressed Up*, which you might also find helpful. Your nearest Disabled Living Centre may have a clothes alteration service or, alternatively, know of someone who can provide this service. (See Appendix 1 for contact details.)

On more general aspects of living alone with Parkinson's, see the PDS information sheet, *Living Alone* (FS29).

My mother, who has had Parkinson's for over 20 years, is beginning to have problems of urinary incontinence and is very distressed by it. What help is available?

Yes, this problem (which may or may not be related to her Parkinson's) is often distressing, but there are things which can be done to help. First you should ask the doctor to examine your mother and identify the cause of the problem as there may be a specific treatment available. There should also be a specialist continence advice service in your mother's local area. Continence advisers are skilled in advising about retraining the relevant muscles, in practical strategies to reduce the likelihood of accidents and in obtaining access to aids and/or laundry services if these become necessary. Your mother's GP surgery should be able to advise you on what is available.

If your mother finds it difficult to talk to her GP about the problems she is having, many continence advisers accept self-referral so you don't have to go through the GP first. The Continence Foundation can provide information on services available in your area. They also provide information, advice and support to people coping with continence problems and have a confidential telephone helpline where it is possible to discuss problems without giving names or feeling embarrassed. You might also find the PDS publication, *Looking After Your Bladder and Bowels in Parkinsonism* (B60) helpful.

10
Eating and diet

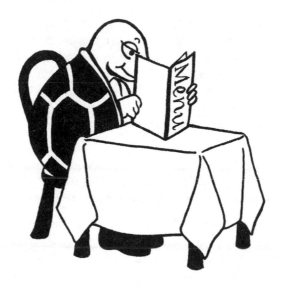

Food, and the way we choose, prepare, present and control it, is a very important part of everyone's life. It can be especially important for people with long-term medical conditions and this is certainly true for people with Parkinson's. When we discussed attitudes in Chapter 5, we stressed the importance of helping yourself, of retaining interests and of feeling in control of your own life. A balanced approach to questions of eating and diet can contribute to all these aims.

Food and drink

What is the recommended diet for people with Parkinson's?

A normal, balanced diet with plenty of high-fibre foods such as wholemeal bread, wholegrain cereals, vegetables (particularly peas and beans), and fresh and dried fruit is recommended. It is also a good idea to drink plenty of fluids – about 8 to 10 cups per day. See the PDS publication *Parkinson's and Diet* (B65).

The Health Development Agency produces attractive, free booklets about various aspects of healthy eating which can be ordered by post (see Appendix 1 for the address) or obtained from your local Centre for Health Promotion/Education if there is one in your area (see under Health in your local phone book for the address and telephone number). There is also a useful paperback called *Cook It Yourself* (details in Appendix 2) which offers some easy suggestions for balanced meals.

I prefer not to take medicines unless absolutely necessary but have quite a lot of trouble with constipation. How can I adjust my diet to help minimize this problem?

Constipation is common in people with Parkinson's and can have several causes. The symptoms can affect bowel muscles and lack of movement or exercise can make the problem worse. Fibre (found in many vegetables, fruits and grains) helps to form soft bulky stools that are easy to pass. Because some people with Parkinson's have trouble chewing and swallowing food, they can find it hard to eat a diet with plenty of fibre. Anticholinergic drugs which are sometimes used to treat Parkinson's can make constipation worse. If the problems are severe, seek advice from your doctor or Parkinson's Disease Nurse Specialist.

Wherever possible, follow the guidelines given in the previous question and be sure to have a breakfast containing wholegrain cereals. Pulses (peas, beans, lentils, etc.), fresh and dried fruit are particularly helpful. It is also important to take a reasonable amount of exercise if you can manage this. If you have problems chewing and swallowing seek advice from a speech and language therapist. A dietitian can provide dietary advice. Do consult your doctor for referral if the problems continue. See the PDS information sheet *Constipation* (FS80).

Can I eat chocolate whilst taking my Parkinson's medication?

Yes. For most people, chocolate creates no specific problems with Parkinson's medication, although we have heard of some individuals who feel that it is unhelpful. Chocolate may be particularly helpful for people who are underweight, although, as with other sweet and sticky foods, you also need to pay careful attention to dental and mouth hygiene.

Is there anything in the idea that eating some kinds of beans can be beneficial?

As mentioned in the answers at the beginning of this chapter, beans are a good source of dietary fibre so in that sense they are helpful. There have also been some reports that broad beans (also known as fava beans) contain levodopa and could be used as a treatment for Parkinson's. Although these beans contain some levodopa, the amount is much less than levodopa tablets such as co-beneldopa (Madopar) and co-careldopa (Sinemet).

There are other concerns about them which are discussed in more detail in the PDS information sheet, *Fava Beans and Parkinson's* (FS55). There have been no comprehensive scientific research trials into these beans and Parkinson's. For all these reasons, they are not considered to be a viable treatment for Parkinson's at the present time. If you want to try these beans it is important that, before doing so, you discuss this with your doctor.

Is it true that foods containing protein can make my wife's Parkinson's worse?

This is an interesting question on a topic about which doctors and researchers are still divided. It is true that protein can interfere with the absorption of levodopa by the brain and thus cause a dose of levodopa taken with or after a protein-rich meal to be less effective. Severe restriction of daytime protein has been tried in people who have serious Parkinson's symptoms and, in some tests, they have shown a marked improvement in response to their levodopa medication.

However, not everyone is helped, the diet is rather unpalatable and therefore difficult for people to sustain, and there are some indications that marked reduction of protein and increase in *carbohydrate* (sugar, bread, pasta, etc.) can lead to more involuntary movements. Another potential complication is that research suggests that people with Parkinson's, especially those with severe muscle rigidity, use up more energy than people of the same age and sex who do not have Parkinson's, and that this may help to account for the excessive weight loss in some people. Restriction of protein intake would make it more difficult to treat such loss of weight.

In general, doctors and dietitians are not in favour of restrictive diets which take away one of life's main pleasures but, for people experiencing major difficulties, a low protein diet (or more simply just eating less protein at one meal) may be worth considering or trying for a while. **However, it should only be undertaken after discussion with the neurologist or other specialist, and under the supervision of a dietitian**. The body needs a certain amount of protein to renew itself and to help it fight infection, so restricting protein may precipitate other problems. See the PDS booklet, *Parkinson's and Diet* (B65) for more information.

What is a normal amount of protein?

It is easier to say what is 'recommended' rather than what is 'normal' because some people in the United Kingdom tend to eat more protein than they need. The amount recommended depends on body weight and is about 0.9 grams per kg of body weight per day. This would mean that a person weighing 70 kg (11 stones) should eat about 60 grams (about 2 oz) of protein per day. However, for all the reasons given in the answer to the previous question, there are other considerations in people with Parkinson's, and reduction or redistribution of protein should only be tried under medical and dietary supervision.

I like a drink (mostly beer) with my friends. Is this all right or will it interfere with my Parkinson's medication?

Alcohol taken in moderation will not interfere with your medication and, if it helps you continue with your normal way of life, it will probably do you good. Obviously everyone, with and without Parkinson's, should avoid excessive drinking. We suggest that you discuss this further with your doctor or Parkinson's Disease Nurse Specialist if you have one.

I have heard that Vitamin B_6 should be avoided by people with Parkinson's. Is this correct?

This vitamin was a potential problem in the early days when levodopa was not combined with a special inhibitor to prevent the levodopa breaking down before it reached the brain. Excessive amounts of Vitamin B_6 made the problem worse. Now that almost everyone takes levodopa preparations such as co-beneldopa (Madopar) and co-careldopa (Sinemet), which contain an inhibitor, there is no problem. Excessive amounts are still best avoided and, if you feel a need for vitamin supplements, you should be able to find some which do not contain vitamin B_6.

Is it true that brown bread contains manganese and that this is a possible cause of Parkinson's and so should be avoided?

It is true that manganese poisoning can cause symptoms similar to those of Parkinson's but this condition is found only in miners in manganese mines and is extremely rare. It is not true that brown or wholemeal breads should be avoided. There is no indication that the ordinary dietary intake of manganese from such foods has any effect on Parkinson's. There is evidence that diets low in fibre are more likely to lead to problems with constipation, a common accompaniment to Parkinson's, so there are definite advantages in eating brown or wholemeal bread.

Eating and swallowing

Eating was one of my mother's main pleasures. Now her tremor and stiffness make mealtimes slow and difficult and she hates to be helped.

Most of us would be very upset if we needed regular help with feeding, so your mother's wish to remain independent is entirely understandable. There are things which can help, although they all require some tolerance of special arrangements and equipment.

Smaller, more frequent meals and snacks of easily managed foods will ease the problem of slowness and special plates to keep food warm can help too. Microwave ovens allow food to be reheated, if it becomes cold and unappetizing. Raising the plate so the distance from plate to mouth is reduced can help to minimize the effects of tremor, as can supporting the elbows on the table. There are many different designs of cutlery and crockery to improve grip and to reduce the likelihood of spillage. These include plate guards, two-handled cups and tumble-not mugs. There are also special eating systems such as the 'Neater Eater' which has a long arm with 'dampers' to reduce the effects of tremor.

The best way to get an assessment of the whole situation, and recommendations especially suitable for your mother, is to contact an occupational therapist through her doctor or social services department (see Chapter 4 for more information on how to make contact). The occupational therapist may suggest a visit to one of the Disabled Living Centres (see Appendix 1 for the Disabled Living Centres Council's address – they will give you details of your nearest centre).

The Disabled Living Foundation also has an information sheet on *Choosing Eating and Drinking Equipment.*

My father has great difficulties in swallowing. What kind of diet should he have to ensure that he gets enough nourishment?

This is a distressing problem found in some people with long-standing Parkinson's. If your father has not been seen by a speech and language therapist to have this problem fully investigated, you should try to arrange this straight away either through self-referral to your local hospital or health board or through your doctor (see Chapter 4 for more information about making contact). The speech and language therapist will be able to suggest some ways of coping with the problems and will also be able to put you in touch with a dietitian who can give specialist advice about adequate nutrition. Meanwhile here are some suggestions:

- **Avoid** mixed textures like liquid with bits such as watery mince and some soups; and flaky or dry foods such as nuts, hard toast and some biscuits.

- **Use** wholemeal bread rather than white bread which tends to form a solid mass and is harder to swallow.

- **Include** some protein-rich foods, such as meat, fish, eggs, cheese and milk, and some energy-rich foods, such as butter, margarine, cream, mayonnaise, sugar, glucose and honey.

- **Purée or thicken** foods to an even consistency. If you purée foods, try to do them separately so that they retain their own colour as it is important that food remains appetizing. Possible thickeners are milk powder, instant potato powder, custard, wholemeal flour, yoghurt, cooked lentils and tinned pease pudding. You could also use a proprietary thickener like Carobel which is obtainable from a chemist. Another option is to use a product called 'Thick and Easy' (available on prescription) which can be used as a thickener and setting agent, but can also be poured over food like bread or cake so that they retain their shape and colour while taking on a different texture. The manufacturers also supply a variety of moulds to help make puréed foods look more like the real thing and so more appetizing.

Are there any other hints to help people with swallowing problems?

Yes there are, but we cannot stress too strongly the need to get expert, individualized advice from a speech and language therapist. Tips to help with swallowing include importance of good posture and taking enough time, also hints such as lowering the chin towards the chest before swallowing, clearing the mouth and throat completely after each bite or spoonful, and sipping very cold fluids before or with meals. See also the question on swallowing in Chapter 3 and the PDS information sheet *Drooling and swallowing* (FS22) for more information.

11
Getting around on wheels

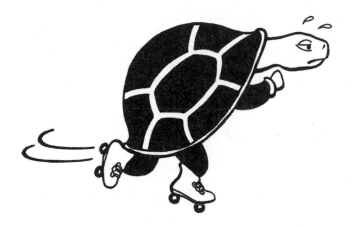

This chapter is all about getting around on wheels – not, we hasten to add, the skates of our intrepid mascot, but the wheels on cars, *pavement vehicles*, scooters and wheelchairs. Although most people with Parkinson's do not use a wheelchair and some have never been car drivers, these are very important topics for those to whom they apply. Most people are car passengers from time to time, so questions about easier entry to and exit from cars may be relevant to anyone with mobility problems.

Almost everyone recognizes the difference that a car can make to their independence and mobility, but wheelchairs are too often seen not as a useful set of wheels but as a symbol of disability. While not in any way wishing to underestimate the distress attached to needing a wheelchair, we do want to encourage the minority of people with Parkinson's who do eventually need a wheelchair to see that using one can widen horizons which may have become very narrow.

For additional information and advice on any of these matters, you can contact the Welfare and Employment Rights Department at the Parkinson's Disease Society who publish an information sheet *Help with Getting Around* (WB 10). The Royal Association for Disability and Rehabilitation (RADAR) publishes information on mobility issues, and Ricability have several reports on various aspects of mobility. Other sources of help include the Disabled Living Foundation, regional Disabled Living Centres and your local DIAL (Disabled Information Advice Line) group. If a telephone number for DIAL does not appear in your local phone book, then DIAL UK, which coordinates the local groups, will be able to provide further information. See Appendix 1 for details.

Getting around without a car

I'm not at all keen on the thought of a wheelchair but my children are urging me to consider having one. How can I discover which type is best for me?

We understand your reluctance to think about a wheelchair. Many people with Parkinson's manage without one for many years after diagnosis, but some people do find them useful if their walking is very unsteady. Some find that they don't need to use a wheelchair all the time, but having one can be useful when they have to travel long distances, if they get tired, or their symptoms are particularly troubling them.

The first approach is to get an assessment to see whether you do need a wheelchair and, if so, whether you need one that is suitable for indoors or outdoors or both. Who provides assessment and advice tends to vary according to the area you live in. However, most statutory provision of wheelchairs is carried out by or though a regional wheelchair service, often based at a local district hospital. Assessment might be provided by a physiotherapist or an occupational therapist. Your doctor should be able to advise further and be able to refer you. Not all types of wheelchair are available on the National Health Service, but an objective assessment will help you to know what choices are available.

Other places that can advise you include the Disabled Living Foundation which has fact sheets on choosing wheelchairs. You could also get advice and try wheelchairs out at one of their Disabled Living Centres. Some of the mobility centres mentioned later on in this chapter also provide advice and assessment on wheelchairs. Some commercial companies that sell specialist equipment, such as Keep Able Ltd, also provide advice and opportunities to try products out before you buy.

Short-term loans can usually be arranged with your local British Red Cross Society, St John Ambulance or Age Concern. Look in your local phone book for the numbers.

Since I gave up driving, I get out of the house much less and I really miss getting around to see old friends, go shopping, etc. I do get a taxi sometimes but it is rather expensive. What else is available?

It is not clear from your question whether your physical condition or finances would allow you to consider having a pavement vehicle of some kind. If so, read the answer to the next question. Otherwise, what is available depends on the area in which you live, but we will mention some of the likely alternatives. Many areas have a special Dial-A-Ride minibus service for people who have mobility problems. You first have to join the scheme – and sometimes there is a waiting list. Once accepted, you can ask the minibus to collect you from your own home and bring you back and the charge is very modest. Some areas have a system of taxi vouchers for people who are unable to take advantage of free or concessionary bus fares. Do enquire about this locally as such schemes can lead to very substantial savings on taxi fares. Citizens Advice or your local authority public transport office should be able to advise further.

While thinking about taxis, it is worth saying – especially to those who used to run their own cars – that you can have a very large number of taxi journeys for what it costs to keep a car on the road. It can be a useful exercise to work out the amounts. If the cost of transport is a problem and you are under retirement age, check if you are eligible for the Mobility Component of the Disability Living Allowance (see the section on *Money and mobility* later in this chapter for more information about this).

For journeys outside your local area, there is an organization called Tripscope (see Appendix 1 for the address) which can help you plan journeys and from which you can also obtain escorts if these are required. Other sources of escorts are the St John Ambulance, the British Red Cross Society and local service organizations such as Rotary, Round Table, Lions and Soroptimists. Your local library or Citizens Advice should be able to provide you with details of the nearest group to you.

See the PDS Welfare and Employment Rights Department information sheet *Help with Getting Around* (WB10*)* for more information.

My walking has been poor for some time and I have an ordinary wheelchair which I can use around the house and which my friends can push when we go out. However, I would like to be more independent and am wondering about a pavement vehicle. How do I go about finding out more?

There are a wide variety of pavement vehicles to suit differing individual needs and different outdoor conditions. As NHS criteria for the issue of outdoor powered vehicles for control by the user are very restrictive, you may need to have funds to pay for your pavement vehicle. It is possible to buy electric wheelchairs as well as cars under the Motability hire purchase scheme (there is a question about Motability in the *Money and mobility* section later in this chapter).

First you need an assessment of the type of vehicle most suited to your needs. As stated in the first question in this section, which focused on wheelchairs, who does the assessment depends on the statutory arrangements in your local area. It will usually be either a physiotherapist or an occupational therapist. You can also visit (by appointment) the Disabled Living Foundation's

Equipment Centre in London or one of the Disabled Living Centres around the country (see Appendix 1 for addresses). Some mobility centres also provide advice on choosing wheelchairs and scooters (see Appendix 1 for contact details). Most commercial suppliers may even make home visits to demonstrate their models (but do not be pressurized into buying without independent advice and time to consider all the options). Some firms supply reconditioned second-hand vehicles. Many specialist magazines and voluntary organization newsletters also carry advertisements for second-hand models.

Pavement vehicles, whether wheelchairs, scooters or buggies can make a major contribution to independence and quality of life. However, they are not cheap, so be sure to try them out and get good advice before deciding to buy.

Can I get any reductions on rail travel?

A disabled person can buy a disabled person's railcard, which will entitle them and an accompanying adult to one third off the price of a rail ticket. Application forms are available from main railway stations or by contacting the Disabled Person's Railcard Office. (See Appendix 1 for contact details.)

Finding accessible toilets is my biggest worry when I am shopping or having a day out. What help is available?

There is a National Key Scheme for Disabled Toilets operated by the Royal Association for Disability and Rehabilitation (RADAR). This is available to anyone who is disabled, by writing to RADAR with the disabled person's name and address plus a declaration in writing confirming their disability (this allows qualification for VAT exemption on the key). A key will be issued costing £3.50 (if you do not qualify for VAT exemption then the key will cost £4.11). A guide to where disabled toilets are located throughout the UK is available from them, price £8.00. (See Appendix 1 for contact details – prices can be subject to change.)

*In*contact, an organization that helps people with continence problems, has produced a 'Just Can't Wait!' card for people who have special toilet needs. This can be shown to staff in high street businesses to gain speedy access to their toilets, or find out about the public toilet facilities in the local area. While it doesn't guarantee access to a shop's toilet, in many cases it will, and at least staff should be able to direct people to the nearest public facilities. (See Appendix 1 for contact details.)

Cars and driving

I like to take my father out shopping or for a drive some-times but getting him in and out of the car is becoming more difficult. Are there ways of easing this problem?

Yes, there are. Which one you choose depends on your father's needs, your particular type of car and how much you want to pay. There is a very simple swivel cushion made by AREMCO (see Appendix 1 for address) which you put on the passenger seat: he will able to swing his legs round into the car much more easily. A plastic bag placed on the seat achieves a similar result.

A less simple, more expensive method is the adaptation or replacement of the whole passenger seat so that it can be turned to face the pavement while the passenger gets in, and then be moved round to the front again once the passenger is seated. If you are changing your car, consider getting one that sits higher off the ground. An occupational therapist or one of the mobility centres mentioned earlier should be able to advise further.

Is it true that I have to notify the DVLA about my Parkinson's?

Yes. Parkinson's is one of a number of medical conditions which can affect driving ability and which therefore have to be notified in writing to the DVLA (the Driver and Vehicle Licensing Agency – see Appendix 1 for the address). They will then send you a PK1 form (Application for a driving licence/notification of driving licence holder's state of health) to fill in and return. For information on what happens after you receive the form, read the answers to the following questions.

Could I lose my driving licence?

You could, but it is unlikely especially if you have only been diagnosed recently. The DVLA will study the information on your completed PK1 (the form mentioned in the answer to the previous question) and, if satisfied that your driving ability is not a hazard to other road users, will issue a three year licence in the majority of cases. At the end of three years, they will review your situation.

The DVLA wants to give drivers with a current or potential disability the best chance of keeping their licences, but it is also responsible for public safety. It is helpful to know how the system works. For example, there are a series of questions on the reverse side of the notification form (PK1) to which you have to answer 'yes' or 'no'. If your answer to any of questions 2–11 is 'yes', you should send a covering letter in which you clarify your answer and explain why you still consider that you are fit to drive. If you do not do this, you may find that your licence is withdrawn unnecessarily.

It is also helpful to discuss your driving ability with your GP and specialist as the DVLA may contact them for their opinions. If there is any disagreement between your doctors and yourself, or if you have some concerns about your driving abilities, it would be worthwhile trying to arrange for an assessment at one of the specialized driving or mobility assessment centres (see Appendix 1 under 'Mobility Assessment Centres' for addresses). There is a question about these centres later in this section.

What does my GP know about my driving ability?

Your GP should know how your medical condition is affecting your use of your hands and legs, and how it could interfere with other faculties like vision which are essential for safe driving – although, even for some of this, he will need good and accurate information from you. Unless he or she has driven down the road behind you, it will not be possible to judge your general driving ability! The variability of Parkinson's itself and, in some people, the unpredictable nature of their response to medication, makes all these judgements more difficult than in some other conditions. That is why it is so important to discuss your driving with your doctor and to request a special *driving assessment* if there is any disagreement or uncertainty.

How do I arrange for a driving assessment?

You should contact your nearest driving assessment centre (see Appendix 1 under 'Mobility Assessment Centres' for how to obtain this information). These are specially staffed and equipped centres around the country which will test your driving capabilities (with adaptations if necessary) and give a report. This report will help you decide whether you want to go on driving, and may be essential evidence if you do lose your licence and want to appeal against the DVLA decision (there is a question about making an appeal later in this section).

There is a charge for these assessments which varies between centres and with the type of assessment required, so it is important to ask for information on charges when you contact the centre.

My driving ability is now rather variable, depending on how I am feeling and how well my tablets are working. I don't want to lose my licence but I don't want to be a danger to myself or other people either. What shall I do?

We sympathize with your dilemma which will be shared by several other people with Parkinson's. However, all drivers have a responsibility to ensure that they are medically fit to drive at all times and to knowingly drive whilst unfit may invalidate insurance cover. You should use your discretion – if in doubt, don't drive. You need to discuss this further with your GP or specialist as soon as possible. An assessment by a mobility centre would also be a good idea. These are listed in the PDS booklet, *Parkinson's and Driving* (B64).

My husband's licence has been withdrawn by the DVLA and he is devastated. We both feel that he is fit to drive – do we have any right of appeal?

Yes, your husband has the right to appeal and, to use it he should write immediately to the DVLA (Driver and Vehicle Licensing Agency) giving notice of his intent to appeal. Even those who are unsure whether to appeal or not are advised to register their intent to do so, as appeals have to be lodged quite soon after notification of the DVLA decision – within six months in England and Wales, and within 21 days in Scotland. The application to appeal can be withdrawn at any time prior to the hearing. All driving licence appeals are heard in the Magistrates' Court (or, in Scotland, in the Sheriffs' Court).

It is extremely difficult to succeed with an appeal unless you have some new evidence – from your doctor or from a driving assessment centre – which was not available at the time of your original application to the DVLA. We would strongly advise that your husband discusses the matter with someone who has special experience in such cases. Possible sources of such advice are your local DIAL (Disability Information Advice Line), or your Citizens Advice. It is very important to be clear about your chance of succeeding with an appeal before going to the hearing because, apart from the distress that an unsuccessful appeal can cause, the DVLA normally seeks to recover its costs (which are likely to be several hundred pounds) if the Court upholds its original decision.

My husband does not want to tell his insurance company about his Parkinson's as he is afraid they will stop him driving. Could they do this?

The answer to this apparently simple question is 'no' and 'yes'. It is not the insurers but the DVLA (Driver and Vehicle Licensing Agency) that is able to decide whether your husband is fit to drive and so may have a driving licence. However, it is illegal to drive on public roads without at least third party insurance, so the insurance company does have some influence on whether a

person is able to drive or not. Your husband **must** notify his
insurance company that he has Parkinson's.

All insurance companies require their clients to tell them the full
facts about any disabilities or serious illnesses that they may have
and about all adaptations made to their cars. Failure to do this will
probably invalidate your husband's insurance. Not only could this
present problems with any claim he might make in the future, it
would also mean that he was driving illegally. The main problem
your husband could face is increased premiums but these are not
inevitable. It is very important to shop around and get several
quotations before making a final decision. It is also essential to
read any potential policy thoroughly, including the small print. By
doing this, your husband will be able to judge what he is getting
for a particular premium. If your husband's present insurance
company increases his premium **because of his Parkinson's**, it
would be worth contacting some of the insurance brokers which
specialize in insuring disabled drivers. There is a list of some of
these companies in *Parkinson's and Driving* (B64) published by
the PDS. We know someone who used one of these specialist
brokers and who paid a lower premium than before his diagnosis!

Money and mobility

Is there any financial support available to help people who have mobility problems?

Yes, though not everyone with mobility problems will be eligible.
There is a Department of Work and Pensions benefit for this
purpose called the Mobility Component of the Disability Living
Allowance (DLA). To be considered for this benefit, applicants
have to be under 65 and they are then assessed against the
disability rules. If they are 'unable or virtually unable to walk
(with aids if used)', they qualify for the higher rate and if they are
'able to walk but need the guidance or supervision of another
person most of the time when walking outdoors', they qualify for
the lower rate.

Obviously there are specific rules and procedures which are difficult to spell out in detail here, so if you think that you may be eligible do telephone or write for a claim pack from the Benefits Agency (the organization that handles social security payments for the Department of Work and Pensions – it will be listed in your local phone book). Try also to discuss the matter with someone knowledgeable like your local DIAL (Disability Information Advice Line) group or the Welfare and Employment Rights Department at the Parkinson's Disease Society (addresses in Appendix 1). The variability of Parkinson's can create particular problems in establishing eligibility for this and other benefits so it is especially important to get advice from an experienced person. There are also review and appeal procedures that you can use if you disagree with the decision made by the adjudication officer or if your circumstances change.

If you have difficulty in filling in forms, get help from a friend or partner.

It is important to establish whether you are eligible for one of the rates of the Mobility Component of DLA because, once granted, they can help you to get other benefits. The rate payable on this Mobility Component can also affect the level of other benefits such as Severe Disablement Allowance, Disability Working Allowance and Disability Premium. There is more information about benefits and other financial issues in Chapter 12 on *Finance*.

Wheelchairs, pavement vehicles, crutches and walking frames are exempt from VAT (Value Added Tax).

What special help is available for drivers?

Those drivers who are granted the higher rate of the Mobility Component (see the answer to the previous question) are eligible for exemption from vehicle excise duty (road tax) on one car. Technically, the vehicle is only exempt when it is being used **'solely by or for the purposes of the disabled person'** but, unless there is flagrant abuse of the exemption, there is unlikely to be any trouble.

People receiving the higher rate of Mobility Component (see the answer to the previous question) are also automatically eligible for a blue badge (previously orange), which confers important parking privileges. They have access to Motability schemes (see the final question in this chapter) and get relief from Value Added Tax on adaptations which make their cars suitable for use by disabled people, and on the installation, repair and maintenance of these adaptations. See the PDS information sheets, *Disability Living Allowance* (WB3) and *Help with Getting Around* (WB10).

Do Mobility Component payments count as income for other purposes such as taxation or means-tested benefits?

No, they are not taxable and should not be considered as income when you are being assessed for other benefits. Nor should any arrears count as capital for means-tested benefits for up to a year after they are paid.

What is Motability?

Motability is a special scheme, available to drivers who have the higher rate of Mobility Component, which helps them to hire, purchase and maintain their cars. It is administered through certain garages and involves handing over the benefit in exchange for certain services, for example having a leased car. For more information you should contact the head office of Motability (see Appendix 1 for the address). See also the Parkinson's Disease Society Information Sheet, *Help with Getting Around* (WB10).

12
Finance

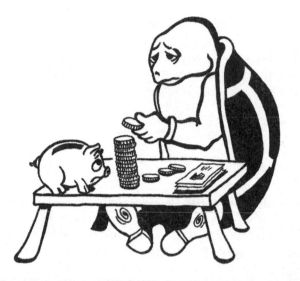

People who have a long-term illness and/or who are elderly often have special needs for treatment, care or equipment. These special needs can significantly increase their living expenses and this is certainly the case for many people with Parkinson's. This chapter provides an outline of some of the main sources of financial support. Other general topics with a financial aspect such as mortgages, insurance policies and prescription charges are also included here, but the money side of motoring is discussed in Chapter 11, and the financial aspects of care outside the home are dealt with in Chapter 13.

This chapter covers a very complex area of knowledge with many detailed rules and allowances for special circumstances.

Not only is it complex, it is also subject to change as the benefits system in this country is reviewed at frequent intervals. People who are in any doubt about their entitlement or who want to question their current levels of financial support will need to make further enquiries. Sources of help include the Department of Work and Pensions, your local Benefits Agency, the local Citizens Advice or your local authority's welfare rights adviser (all of these organizations should be listed in your local phone book). You can also contact the Welfare Benefits and Employment Rights Department at the Parkinson's Disease Society (address in Appendix 1) who produce information sheets on benefits and employment issues affecting people with Parkinson's. All of these people and organizations should also be able to provide information about the current levels of various benefits.

Benefits

I am 36, single and over the last few months have been either unemployed (I lost my job six months ago) or off sick (when control of my Parkinson's symptoms causes trouble). I am finding it increasingly difficult to manage financially – what help is available to me?

A combination of unemployment and the fluctuating nature of your Parkinson's has placed you in a difficult position. You should certainly talk to your doctor about the chances of improving the control of your Parkinson's, and to a disability employment adviser at your local Jobcentre Plus about employment and/or retraining possibilities (you will find more information about this in the section on *Work* in Chapter 8).

If you have enough National Insurance Contributions to your credit, you should currently be receiving either Incapacity Benefit (if you have been off sick for more than 28 weeks) or Contribution-based Jobseekers Allowance (if you are currently registered as unemployed). Neither of these benefits is means-tested. If they are insufficient to meet your needs, you can apply to be assessed for Income Support, which is means-tested, but which, if granted, carries automatic access to some other benefits like free prescriptions, free dental treatment, vouchers for spectacles and other appliances, and housing benefit and council tax rebates.

If you do not have sufficient National Insurance contributions to your credit, you may be receiving income-based Jobseekers Allowance or Income Support.

If you return to work but at relatively low rates of pay, you may be entitled to the Working Tax Credit. There are both advantages and disadvantages vis-à-vis other entitlements if you return to work and claim this new benefit (for more details see the next question), so you should be sure to talk to someone who can help you do this calculation. There should be a nominated person in each Benefits Agency or Jobcentre Plus office who can give you information, or you could approach one of the organizations or people mentioned in the introduction to this chapter. You will find social security offices listed under 'Benefits Agency' in your local phone book, while Jobcentre Plus offices will be listed under 'Employment Service' or you can find your nearest one using their website. See Appendix 1 for contact details.

What is the Working Tax Credit?

As of April 2003, this benefit has replaced the Disabled Person's Tax Credit. It is a payment to top up the earnings of working people on low incomes, including those who do not have children. There are extra amounts for working households in which someone has a disability. People without children claim Working Tax Credit if they are 16 years or over and have a disability such as Parkinson's that puts them at a disadvantage in getting a job. It is available to employees and self-employed people and includes support for the costs of qualifying childcare. You cannot receive Working Tax Credit if you are not working. You have to be over 16 years of age, work 16 hours or more in paid work and expect to work for at least 4 weeks. In addition you have to either responsible for one child or have a disability which puts you at a disadvantage in getting a job.

Claim forms are available from the Inland Revenue – See Appendix 1 for contact details. See also the PDS Welfare Benefits information sheet *Working Tax Credit* (WB4) for more information.

What is the Disability Living Allowance and who can claim it?

The Disability Living Allowance is a non-means-tested benefit paid to people under 65 at the time of application, who require personal care or supervision by day or night and/or to people who have considerable mobility problems. It has separate care (three levels) and mobility (two levels) components so people with a wide range of different needs may be eligible. Application forms can be obtained by ringing the Benefits Agency free phone number 0800 88 22 00 or from the Welfare Benefits and Employment Rights Department at the Parkinson's Disease Society (address in Appendix 1). If you intend to ask your GP or other health professional to write their comments on your application form, it is good idea to ask their opinion about your eligibility beforehand. Get help with filling in the form if you have difficulty. See the PDS Welfare Benefits information sheet *Disability Living Allowance* (WB3) for more information.

My father has received the lower rate of Attendance Allowance for the past two years but now needs more supervision. Can he apply for the higher rate and how is the decision made?

Attendance Allowance is for people aged 65 and over at the time of application, who need a lot of care or supervision. If circumstances change, he (or you on his behalf) can apply for a review at any time. Just write to the Disability Benefits Unit (see Appendix 1 for contact details) with an explanation of the change in circumstances. Your letter will be acknowledged and they will make various enquiries to establish whether or not he is entitled to the higher rate. These enquiries could include letters to your father; to his doctor or consultant; and, in some cases, a special medical examination.

You are more likely to succeed with your claim if you get help and advice from someone with previous experience of such applications, such as the PDS Welfare and Employment Rights Department. People applying for this benefit for the first time are also advised to obtain some expert help in completing the application form.

We applied for Attendance Allowance for my wife but were refused. Is it worth appealing?

If you feel that you have a case, it is certainly worth pursuing the matter, as some applications which fail the first time are granted on review. Please read the answer to the previous question and try to obtain some expert help in completing the form. It is easy with something variable like Parkinson's to give an unrealistically optimistic picture of the situation.

I do not live with my elderly mother-in-law but I share the task of caring for her with my sister-in-law. She gets the Carers' Allowance – is it possible that I could be eligible too?

No, only one person can claim the Carers' Allowance for a particular disabled person but, if you are spending a minimum of 35 hours per week looking after your mother-in-law, you can claim Home Responsibilities Protection for each full year spent caring. This can help to protect your own pension rights so it is worth applying. The PDS Welfare and Employment Rights Department information sheets on *the Carers Allowance* (WB8) and *Welfare Benefits General Information* (WB1) which cover Home Responsibilities Protection.

Is there any help available with the cost of prescriptions for Parkinson's drugs?

The disappointing answer to this question is 'no' – there is no specific exemption because of a diagnosis of Parkinson's, although the PDS has been fighting for such an exemption for many years. However, many people with Parkinson's qualify for exemption from prescription charges on general grounds such as being over pensionable age or being in receipt of Income Support or being unable to collect their prescriptions themselves. See the PDS information sheet *National Health Service Costs* (WB9*)*, which is available from the PDS Welfare and Employment Rights Department, for more details.

This still leaves some younger people with Parkinson's, often on low incomes, struggling with heavy prescription costs. The only partial relief available in this situation is to pre-pay for your prescriptions by purchasing a *season ticket*, which can last for either four or 12 months and covers all the drugs you need during that period, not just the drugs for your Parkinson's. To apply, you need to fill in form FP95 (in England), EC05 (in Scotland) available from most doctors' surgeries, from pharmacists, from Post Offices, or from the Health Authority. Before you go ahead, you need to do a careful calculation, based on the current price of ordinary prescriptions, the price of season tickets and your average number of prescriptions in a year, to see whether a season ticket will be helpful to you. Some GPs will prescribe larger quantities in one go.

Other financial considerations

I was just about to buy a house when I was told I had Parkinson's. Will I be able to get a mortgage?

As with all decisions about mortgages, the answer will depend on your personal circumstances including your savings, income, likely security of employment (which may be affected by the diagnosis of Parkinson's) and on how much you want to borrow. Once you are sure in your own mind that you want to go ahead, you should shop around to see what various building societies and banks have on offer. The PDS Welfare and Employment Rights Department produces an information sheet *Pensions, Insurance and Independent Financial Advice* (WB15), which may be helpful.

What attitude do life insurance companies take to a diagnosis of Parkinson's?

Life insurance companies normally ask people who wish to take out new policies to answer questions about their health or to undergo a medical examination. If these reveal a long-term condition like Parkinson's, the result can be either refusal or high premiums. However, there have recently been some widely publicized 'Over-50s' insurance schemes which guarantee acceptance without a medical or any questions. The benefits at death (after the first two years) are relatively small fixed amounts, so if you live for many years, you could end up paying in more than the guaranteed benefit. You would, however, have several years of security, so such schemes may be worth considering, if you feel that you are underinsured.

On the other hand, people with long-term medical conditions may get more favourable rates when it comes to buying an annuity, because, on average, the insurers will assume that they will live for fewer years after retirement. However, all annuities and pensions involve complex calculations and weighing up of options, so it is very important to get the advice of an independent financial adviser. The PDS Welfare and Employment Rights Department produces an information sheet *Pensions, Insurance and Independent Financial Advice* (WB15), which may be helpful.

I am 55, married with a wife and two teenage children. I am considering retiring from work because of ill health. What are the main economic factors that I should consider in making my decision?

You have not told us what your work is or which aspect of your Parkinson's is causing you to consider this course of action, so we can only give a general outline of the main considerations for anyone in this position. The important thing is not to rush into anything and to get as much information as possible about the choices open to you and about your likely sources of income.

First you need to consider whether you may, either now or in the future, consider a different kind of work. This might be full or part-time and would be an especially important consideration for someone further away than you are from statutory retirement age. If this seems relevant, you should discuss the principle of other kinds of work and how these might affect your health with your GP. If some alternative type of work is a likely option, then we would suggest you read the section on *Work* in Chapter 8.

Secondly you need to consider the practical route by which your retirement can be achieved. Once you and your GP are agreed that your health problems mean that you will be physically or mentally incapable of further work, you need to discover how the arrangements for your retirement can be made and how they will affect your future income.

If you have any doubts about your employer's attitude, it may be best to start with your union or professional body. If you are not a member of such an organization, you could contact your local Citizens Advice (see your local phone book for the address and telephone number). Although most employers are helpful, do remember that, irrespective of any health problem, you have the right not to be unfairly dismissed. If you have been continually employed by your present employer for two years or more, you have the right to pursue any dissatisfaction about the manner in which your employment ends through an industrial tribunal.

Assuming that your employer is one of the many who are helpful, you should discuss the matter with him or her. In many instances, early retirement can be arranged with their full cooperation and support. Where occupational pension schemes are involved, they may, for example, assist employees to decide the most favourable route and timing for retirement. Details of any company pension scheme are usually available from your personnel department or directly from the pension company.

Thirdly you need to consider the full financial implications of giving up work. Your present and future financial commitments will be one part of the calculation, as will the question of whether your wife goes out to work or may do so in the future. If you have an occupational pension, you will still be eligible for the various non-means-tested benefits. Then, depending on your contributions record and degree of disability, you may be eligible for Incapacity Benefit (although, even with the support of your doctor, it is difficult to be absolutely certain of this) or Disability Living Allowance (see the section on **Benefits** earlier in this chapter for more information about these).

If you are not eligible for an occupational pension, then you may be eligible for some means-tested benefits such as Income Support, Housing Benefit and Council Tax Benefit. Eligibility for Income Support opens up access to other sorts of help such as free prescriptions, free dental treatment and free school meals for your children. Every type of benefit has its own qualifying conditions so it is very important to seek advice about the likely situation for your own individual circumstances. This can be obtained from the Benefits Agency, Citizens Advice (see your local phone book for address and phone numbers for both organizations), a welfare rights office (check with your local authority) or from the Welfare and Employment Rights Department at the PDS (see Appendix 1 for the address and phone number). The PDS Welfare and Employment Rights Department produces an *Employment Pack* which includes information on the issue of early retirement on health grounds.

Can I get financial assistance from anywhere other than the Benefits Agency?

You may be able to get assistance for specific purposes such as help with the purchase of a particular item of equipment or a holiday from funds held by trade unions, professional organizations, the benevolent funds of services (the army, navy and air force), local and national charitable trusts, churches and so on. The range of possible sources and of the conditions placed on recipients of grants varies enormously but usually you have to establish some personal connection. Your local library may have the *Charities Digest* (see Appendix 2) which lists many of these funds, and some Councils of Voluntary Service now have computer programs that can save you time by helping to identify the most likely sources for any particular set of circumstances. (If there is nothing listed under Council of Voluntary Service in your local phone book, the National Association of Councils for Voluntary Service can tell you whether there is one in your area [see Appendix 1 for contact details]. If there isn't one in your area, then ask at your local Citizens Advice about any local groupings of voluntary organizations which may be able to help in this way.) These organizations and your local library may also have a copy of a directory called *A Guide to Grants for Individuals in Need* (see Appendix 2 for details). It contains a comprehensive list of organizations which can provide funds and the circumstances in which they might do so.

The Disabled Living Foundation publishes a fact sheet, *Sources of Funding and Obtaining Equipment for Disabled and Older People*, which can be downloaded from their website or ordered by post. The Directory of Social Change produces a directory, *A Guide to Grants for Individuals in Need*, which contains a list of organizations that will give grants and funding. There is also an organization called Charity Search, which provides information on sources of funding for older people. See Appendix 1 for contact details and Appendix 2 for details of how to obtain these publications.

As mentioned in the section on **Work** in Chapter 8, equipment to help you obtain or retain employment is also available from the Department of Work and Pensions, as is contribution to the cost of journeys to work. The local Jobcentre Plus can advise further. See Appendix 1 for contact details.

My husband is becoming very confused and is now unable to handle his financial affairs. Is there some way that I can be authorized to act for him?

This is quite a complex area of the law, and we would recommend that you discuss your situation with someone at Citizens Advice. (See Appendix 1 for contact details.) They will be able to tell you if you need advice from a solicitor. Before you take any action, you may find it useful to read Age Concern's *Factsheet No.22: Legal Arrangements for Managing Financial Affairs*. There is a version for England and Wales, and another – with the same number – for Scotland (where the law is different). You can obtain copies from the relevant Age Concern offices (the addresses and phone numbers are in Appendix 1). Carers UK have a booklet (free to carers) called *Dealing with Someone Else's Money* (see Appendix 2 for details). All these publications set out the various options ranging from simple permissions to cash social security benefits to the legal documents required in cases of proven mental incapacity.

If your husband still has times when he is able to understand what he is doing, then you should discuss with him as soon as possible the idea of making an Enduring Power of Attorney. This is a legal document which allows him to appoint one or more persons to act for him. The document has to be drawn up on a special form and signed by both the donor (your husband) and the attorney (yourself and any others he appoints – the 'attorney' in a Power of Attorney does not mean a lawyer, although he could appoint a solicitor as his attorney if he wished to do so). It has to be completed while your husband is able to understand what he is signing. If he then becomes incapable of managing his own affairs, you apply to the Court of Protection (part of the Supreme Court) for registration of your Power of Attorney and you are then authorized to act for him without his consent. While you are organizing your Power of Attorney you could also encourage your husband to make a will if he has not already made one.

If your husband is already too confused to understand what is involved in making an Enduring Power of Attorney, you will have to apply to the Court of Protection to be appointed as a Receiver (or, in Scotland, a Curator Bonum) for your husband's affairs. This is a more complex and costly procedure than making a Power of Attorney so it is certainly advisable to act sooner rather than later if at all possible.

13
Care outside the home

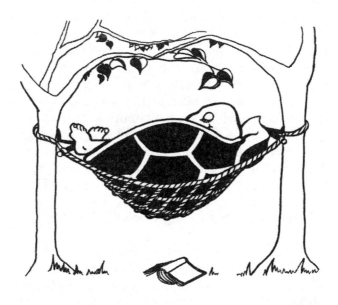

As with most other sections of the population, the vast majority of people with Parkinson's spend most of their time at home. However, sometimes, from choice or necessity, they spend some time outside the home. This chapter is about the variety of circumstances and locations in which this can occur. Except for holidays or respite care facilities that cater for couples, most of these situations involve the separation of the person with Parkinson's from their carer and so can create anxieties for both parties. People differ greatly in their needs and choices and the range of provision can vary from one area to another – our answers can only indicate the likely solutions and suggest ways of following them up.

Respite care

What is respite care?

Respite care is any facility or resource that allows those who care for sick, frail, elderly or disabled relatives or friends to have a break from their caring tasks. We have discussed some of the 'in-house' aspects of respite care in Chapter 5, so this section will concentrate on breaks outside the home. Such breaks do not come as a right as holidays do with a paid job but they are equally, if not more, important and necessary. Awareness of this need is, however, growing, and the National Strategy for Carers launched in early 1999 was an important sign of government recognition.

Carers UK publish a leaflet, *Taking a Break* and the PDS has an annual guide to facilities for both respite care and holidays called *Holidays and Respite Care* (B66).

I don't want to go away but would like the occasional day or half-day to recharge my batteries and keep me sane. Do you know anywhere I can get this?

In the chapter on *Caring for the 'carers'* in Chapter 6, we discussed how help could be brought into the home through schemes like Crossroads – Caring for Carers. Such schemes are, of course, an important way of having a break, although they tend to be for a few hours rather than a whole day.

You should contact your social services department to see what sort of respite services they offer. Some have Family Link schemes whereby another family will agree to take your relative into their home on a regular basis – for a few hours, a day, a weekend or even longer. All social services departments have some day centres offering company, meals, activities and supervision; they will also know about any similar facilities in your area provided by voluntary organizations such as the Red Cross and the Women's Royal Voluntary Service. Day centres cannot usually cope with severely disabled people, but there are other choices such as day hospitals (especially if some re-assessment or treatment is required) and day care in residential or nursing homes.

An approach via social services would be a useful first step, as they will assess the needs of your relative and yourself, take into account your preferences, and suggest what is available as well as providing details of what it will cost. Perhaps you should not exclude the possibility of a longer break which could be good for both of you. It will not hurt to know what is available.

I really want to continue looking after my wife, but feel the need for regular breaks to keep me going. What is available?

Regular breaks can make an important contribution to people's ability to go on caring for their relatives. One major determinant of what is available is the type of care that your wife needs. If she does not require skilled nursing or special equipment, she may be able to have a regular break (how often depends on your needs and local resources) in a local authority or private residential home. If you think this is likely to be a suitable solution, approach your social services department with your request. They should assess your situation and tell you what is available to meet your needs. If your need is very urgent, your choice of places may be very restricted; with more time to plan, you will probably have some choice. There will be a charge related to your ability to pay.

If your wife is severely disabled and needs nursing care, you may be able to arrange for her to go into hospital (usually in the care of a geriatrician), or (in some areas) into a local authority-funded bed in another place like a nursing home, while you have a break. Depending on the level of need and the availability of local resources, the frequency of such admissions can vary from once a year up to every few weeks. You need to ask your GP if you want this kind of respite care. There is no charge for hospital or local authority-funded care but, in some circumstances, benefits and allowances may be affected.

I don't know what to do. I am at my wits' end and feel in need of a break but my husband gets upset if I mention it, and I am not sure that anyone else could look after him properly anyway.

Your distress and ambivalent feelings are shared by many people who have been caring for a relative for many years and are entirely understandable – as is your husband's anxiety about being cared for by someone else. It is a start to have put your feelings into words and now you need someone with whom you can explore them further. It will help if this person is someone who understands about Parkinson's and who also knows what options are open to you. You could talk to your doctor, to someone from social services, a Parkinson's Disease Nurse Specialist, a community nurse or, if there is a local PDS branch nearby, one of their community support workers. If you prefer to discuss your needs and ideas on the telephone, you could use the PDS's confidential Helpline. You are almost certainly correct in thinking that no one will be able to look after your husband as well as you do but, by having a break, you will probably be able to carry on caring for him for longer, which is what you both want. You may also find that your husband is quite worried about you and that it will be easier for him to think through the problem if someone else is involved in the discussions. Try to find out as much as you can about any places that are suggested and visit them if at all possible. In this way, you can see for yourself what standard of service is being offered. If you decide after all to go somewhere together, the PDS's Holidays and *Respite Care Guide* (B66), published annually, has a section on respite or holidays with care facilities. See also Chapter 6 – *Caring for the 'carers'*.

Both my mother and I would really like a break. Is there anywhere we can go so that we both get a break but don't have to be separated?

Yes, the publication mentioned at the end of the previous answer will give you various options in different parts of the country. If your mother is well enough to have a holiday rather than respite care, then we suggest that you also read the next section on *Holidays*.

Holidays

My husband and I have not had a holiday for years because of my Parkinson's – really I have lost confidence. Could you suggest anything which would be suitable?

It is easy to lose confidence when you have not been away for a long time but take courage in both hands because there are a whole range of possibilities. First you need to decide between yourselves what sort of holiday you would like and how far you want to travel. Think about how much care and attention you need and whether you want to have access to particular activities or pastimes. The PDS publishes an annual *Holidays and Respite Care Guide* (B66), which provides information on short stays, respite care and holidays for people with Parkinson's, their carers and families.

Other organizations that provide information and advice about holidays for people with special needs are the Holiday Care Service, which can suggest particular places and advise about transport, insurance and people to contact for help in meeting the cost of a holiday; and RADAR (Royal Association for Disability and Rehabilitation), which produces very informative guides on holidays in the British Isles and abroad.

If you have a particular resort in mind, it would be worth contacting their tourist information office, as many holiday resorts produce special information about accommodation and facilities for people with disabilities. Your local social services department may also have some general information. In some towns there are travel agents or coach operators who offer special holidays for people with mobility problems, so do ask around to find out if there is something like this in your locality. Some local PDS branches also organize weekend or longer holidays.

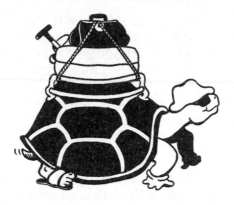

The Winged Fellowship Trust, a charity committed to providing real holidays for people with disabilities, has purpose-built or specially adapted holiday homes, which can cater for people with severe mobility problems. Partners, relatives or friends, who would normally care for the person, can also go on the holiday, but the Winged Fellowship Trust employ experienced care staff, and recruit young volunteers to help to look after the holiday-makers so that the 'carer' has a holiday too. Another organization is the Calvert Trust, which runs holiday centres for people with disabilities and their families. (See Appendix 1 for details of these organizations.)

If you are going abroad, either on an organized holiday or independently, remember to arrange adequate insurance cover (and to tell the insurance company about your Parkinson's). Medical attention is free in all European Union countries although you should obtain form number E111 (from the Post Office) before you go. The PDS information sheet *International Travel and Parkinson's* (FS28) has more tips on travelling abroad.

I need to get away for a break but would feel happier if my father, who has Parkinson's, could have a holiday rather than just go into a hospital or a home. What can you suggest?

Most of the organizations mentioned in the answer to the previous question cater for people on their own. The Winged

Fellowship was founded to provide just the sort of thing you are looking for – a break for you and a real holiday for your father. With their holidays you can either go with your father, but care can be provided so that you have a holiday as well, or your father can go on his own. If your father has a holiday in mind but needs someone to go with him, The Holiday Care Service has an information guide on *Escorts and Carers*, which you might find useful.

I would love a holiday but don't think that I could afford anywhere with the special facilities I need. Are there any sources of financial help?

Yes there are, although your eligibility for help will depend on your personal circumstances. The Holiday Care Service (address in Appendix 1) can put enquirers in touch with possible sources of financial help. Some towns have charitable funds for use by local residents (ask at your local authority offices or local library), and there are a large number of benevolent funds listed in two books, which we have already mentioned in Chapter 12 – the *Charities Digest* and *A Guide to Grants for Individuals in Need* (your local library or Citizens Advice should have reference copies).

Going into hospital

My wife has to go into hospital shortly. Her speech is now very indistinct and she is used to having me on hand all day. I understand her needs and what she can and cannot do. Is there some way I can pass on this information without seeming to interfere?

Going into hospital creates anxiety for most people even if they are able to communicate easily, so you are very wise to think ahead about your wife's special needs.

The PDS publishes information sheets on *Going into Hospital* (FS61), which includes information and issues to consider when

Information for Use on Admission to Hospital or Respite Care

If you have Parkinson's and are to be admitted to hospital or having respite care, you may find it helpful to complete this form, giving details of your drug regime and other relevant information which you consider would be helpful to the nursing staff responsible for your care.

Name: _____ Date: _____

The following drug(s) have been prescribed.

NB: It is important that they are taken at the times indicated.

Drug name	Dose	Time

Activity	Assistance Required/Aids Used
Speech	
Comprehension	
Eating/Drinking	
Walking	
Washing/Bathing	
Dressing	
Turning Over In Bed	
Bowels/Bladder	
Other Information	

Figure 13.1 Information form for use on admission to hospital or respite care

going into hospital. It includes a simple form (Figure 13.1), which you can complete and give to staff at a pre-assessment clinic or when your wife is admitted to hospital. Keep a copy on you for any new staff you meet. Many hospitals now have a named nurse allocated to each patient, and it would obviously be a good idea to discuss the completed form with the named nurse when your wife is admitted. There is a companion information sheet for professionals, which discusses some of the particular concerns that they should be aware of when someone with Parkinson's is admitted to hospital or for respite care. This is called *Hospital Stays and Parkinson's Disease* (FS62).

If your wife uses a portable communication aid, make sure that she takes it with her into hospital and let the staff know that she uses it. A speech and language therapist in the hospital could also advise further. If there is a Parkinson's Disease Nurse Specialist available, ask him or her to talk to the staff to prepare them for your stay.

I have to go into hospital soon for an operation and need my Parkinson's medication at irregular hours. I would feel much less anxious if I knew that I could keep my tablets and take them when I need them. Will this be allowed or can they insist that I hand them over?

Your anxiety is shared by many people with Parkinson's who know only too well that sometimes even a few minutes can make a big difference. Some hospital wards, especially non-neurological wards, are not generally geared up for people with very individual medication timetables and there have been many accounts of problems arising from this. However, there is a growing awareness of the serious difficulties that standard drug rounds (when nurses give out medication at set times and not otherwise) cause for people with Parkinson's. Some hospital wards allow self-medication, and others provide a more individualized approach to medication timings. You should discuss your wish to retain control of your medication with the hospital consultant and the ward sister, and see if you can come to a satisfactory arrangement. Make sure that they understand the importance of having your drugs at the individual times to suit you as they may not be aware of this unless they specialize in Parkinson's. If you have a Parkinson's Disease Nurse Specialist, discuss your concern with them as they may be able to liaise with the hospital staff. Take copies of the PDS information sheets *Going into Hospital* (FS61) and *Hospital Stays and Parkinson's Disease* (FS62) (mentioned in the previous question) with you.

Some simple advice from a Parkinson's Disease Nurse Specialist (L. Macnamara [letter]. *Parkinson* 2003 [Spring]: 23), includes:

- Always carry with you a couple of notes of your medication regime, not just the names but the exact doses and times, in case of emergency.

- Don't assume that the doctors and nurses will know what you take and which times suit you best. You may know more about Parkinson's than they do.

- When you are admitted to hospital, give a note to the doctor who writes up the medicine chart.

- Stick another note to the front or top of your bedside locker.

- Ask that your named nurse writes the times of your medication and the reason for the times as part of your care plan.

- If your medication is not given correctly without proper explanation, ask for your concern to be documented in that care plan.

- You may feel a nuisance or get worked up if you or a relative repeatedly remind staff but try to keep calm. Persistence will pay off.

- If things are still not working, arrange an interview with the named nurse, the ward manager or the doctor. This is better than trying to grab them when they are busy. Each ward has a pharmacist too, usually based in the main pharmacy department: ask to speak to them.

- If you are too ill to do all this, make sure a friend or relative knows what to do for you.

- If staff do get it right, please compliment them, and write to the hospital managers when you get home. By highlighting good practice, we can ensure that it is spread.

See also the next question on anaesthesia.

My wife is due to go into hospital for a hysterectomy and I am worried because I have heard that the anaesthetic may upset her Parkinson's medication. Is this true and can anything be done to prevent it?

It is not so much that the anaesthetic 'upsets' the Parkinson's medication as that operations under anaesthetic require that anything taken by mouth (food or drink or medicine) has to be withdrawn shortly before the operation. This causes very understandable anxiety to people like your wife who depend on their medication for reasonable mobility and comfort.

Do talk to the medical, surgical and nursing staff on her ward so that they understand how important your wife's Parkinson's medication is, and that it needs to be withdrawn for the shortest possible time. If there is a local Parkinson's Disease Nurse Specialist, you could perhaps ask her to liaise with the staff on the ward. Nowadays, anaesthetists encourage their patients to take all essential medication up to the time of the operation. Essential medicines include those for Parkinson's, high blood pressure and steroids.

Apomorphine (Apo-go), which is given by injection, can sometimes be used to provide some relief from symptoms until the usual drug regimen can be resumed. If your wife is on a complicated drug regimen, it is likely that apomorphine will provide some control over her symptoms, but this will not be at the same level as she is used to. To use apomorphine, it is necessary for the antisickness drug, domperidone (Motilium), to be given before the operation. However, this drug can be given by suppository, so it could be used if she has to be 'nil by mouth'. If your wife is already on apomorphine, she should be able to continue taking it throughout the period before, during and after the operation.

See the PDS information sheet, *Anaesthesia and Parkinson's* (FS36) for more information. Also see the previous question for general information on going into hospital.

My husband (aged 79 and suffering from Parkinson's) was poorly treated and neglected whilst in hospital recently. How can I complain?

We are very sorry to learn of your husband's unhappy experience and would certainly encourage you to make a complaint.

All hospitals (and social services departments) now have to have complaints procedures and to make them known to the public. Many have special leaflets which set out what action you should take and whom you can contact, either to make the complaint yourself or to get help and support in making it.

In general, our advice would be that, if you are concerned about any aspect of health service provision, then you should discuss your concern, as soon as possible, with the person who gave (or failed to give) the service in question. Sometimes misunderstandings or disagreements can be sorted out in this direct face-to-face way. If you are nervous or uncertain, take a friend or relative with you.

If this action leaves you dissatisfied, ask to speak to the Patient Advice and Liaison Services (PALS) Officer at the hospital. This officer will listen to your concerns and help to ensure that the relevant people are involved. He or she will also help you to get in touch with an independent advocate should you wish to proceed further with your complaint. An advocate will understand how the complaint system works and will help you to think through your options, prepare your evidence and, if you wish, arrange for someone to accompany you at meetings with hospital managers. See Chapter 4 for more information about the role of the PALS.

Do not be afraid to make your complaint. Even though your husband's unhappy experience cannot be changed now, you can alert the hospital to the problem and so help to improve standards for other users. There are three golden rules for anyone wanting to make a complaint: complain as soon as possible after the incident, be courteous, and provide accurate details of the incident such as date, time, place and people involved.

See the PDS publication, *Choices: using and understanding health and social care* (B70). Counsel and Care, an organization that provides information and advice to older people, also has an information sheet *Making a Complaint about Community Care and NHS Services* (Factsheet No. 18), which you might find helpful.

My father is in hospital and I am worried that they will discharge him without sufficient help. He lives near me but is unrealistic about what he can do for himself. I supervise and do some meals but can only do a certain amount because I also have to care for my disabled husband. What should I do?

Mention your concerns to the ward sister immediately and ask to see a social worker. Since April 1993, every hospital and its local social services department has had to have an approved hospital discharge agreement. This is meant to ensure that people like your father are not sent back home without adequate services.

If he has complex needs, he should receive a full community care assessment (see Chapter 4 for more information about these) which should also include an assessment of your needs as his carer. Ask specifically for such an assessment if it is not offered. Stick to your guns and insist that he is given this assessment. Remember that you also have the right to comment on its findings. If the result of the assessment is a recommendation for residential or nursing home care, there is further relevant information in the next section.

Counsel and Care have an information sheet called *Hospital Discharge and Continuing Care in England* (Factsheet No. 13) which you might find useful.

Long-term care

How do I find the right residential or nursing home accommodation for my needs?

First you need to be sure what your needs are and whether you want to opt for permanent care outside your own home. Knowing the type of care you require will help you to decide whether you could remain at home if you wished to do so or, if you could not, whether you need residential home or nursing home care. Another important element in the equation is your age and whether or not you have a spouse who also has some care needs. Do try to talk the whole question over from every possible angle with someone you trust – deciding on permanent care is a very important decision and not one to be taken lightly.

If you have family and friends near your present home, you will probably want to stay in the same area. Unless you are able to pay the full cost of your care for several years, you will need your local social services to agree that you are in need of long-term care. You should therefore contact the department and ask for an assessment. They will provide a written report, an assessment of your needs and the options for meeting them, with which you can agree or disagree.

Whether you need financial assistance or not, you need to find out what is available. Your local social services department and Primary Care Trust will have lists of all registered homes in the area and some information about size and facilities. However, there is no substitute for visiting the homes and seeing things for yourself. Do ask questions (see the next answer for some suggestions) – of the staff, of the residents and of their relatives. Local professional workers and volunteers may also have useful comments and experiences to add to your own researches.

If, alternatively, you want to move to another part of the country, perhaps to be near a relative, you need to make the same sort of enquiries in that area. If you are likely to need financial assistance, you will still have to involve the social services department for the place where you live now.

In circumstances where the type or quality of care is more important than its location – perhaps because you are relatively young or have particular problems in controlling your Parkinson's symptoms – there are a few other options. One might be a home like those owned and run by the Leonard Cheshire Foundation which tend to have younger residents. Nearly all such homes have waiting lists and you will need to take this into account when making your plans. See the PDS publication *Choices* (B70) for more information.

What sort of questions should I have in mind when viewing a residential or nursing home?

Just as in thinking about moving to a new house, the potential list of questions is very long indeed! We have tried to highlight a few key areas.

The first crucially important questions are about the type and quality of medical, nursing and specialist care available. This will relate mainly to your present needs, but it will be worth enquiring what will happen if you need additional care in the future. You may want to know whether you can keep your own doctor (if he or she is willing to visit) and whether dentists, opticians and therapists make regular visits to the home.

Secondly you need to consider the nature and quality of the accommodation. You could ask questions about its overall size, whether there is a choice of single or shared rooms, the availability of sitting and recreation rooms, the standard and variety of washing and bathroom facilities, ease of access including ramps and lifts, and whether there are special arrangements or rules about smoking or pets.

Your third area of interest is the general atmosphere. Are the staff welcoming but also open to questions? Do the other residents look well cared for, comfortable and interested in what is going on? Is there sufficient privacy? Are there facilities for visitors to stay overnight?

Location is another important topic. If you wish to remain in the area that you know well, in order to keep in touch with family, friends, particular facilities like church, shops or meeting places, then this will be a crucial consideration for you. Alternatively you may wish to move to another district or town to be close to relatives or friends, or you may wish to live in a particular home where you already have friends or contacts. On a more general level, you may prefer a quiet, rural location or a busy, urban one.

The PDS publication *Choices* (B70) has a checklist of questions and points to consider when visiting any potential homes. You may also find Counsel and Care's *What to Look For in a Care Home* (Factsheet No. 19) helpful. Counsel and Care is an organization that provides information and advice to older people (see Appendix 1 for contact details).

What if the place I like charges more than I can afford from my own income?

If your income and savings are greater than the maximum allowed under current government regulations (you can check what this is by contacting your local social services department or Benefits Agency) then you would not be eligible for help from social services. In these circumstances you would have to see if what you can afford in fees could be topped up from elsewhere – for example by a relative, or by a grant from a charity or benevolent fund on which you have some call. If, on the other hand, your income and capital are below the cut-off level, and you have been assessed as needing the type of care provided by this particular home, and the costs do not exceed those normally allowed by social services for such care, then any shortfall will be met by the social services department.

If you have a home to sell and you are going into permanent residential care, you can use the capital or interest from investments to pay the costs.

The social services department, or the Citizens Advice will be able to offer more specific advice related to your individual circumstances.

My father was taken into hospital after a fall when he broke his hip. He is now very confused and I am told that he must go into a private nursing home. Can they do this?

Before considering permanent care it is important to find out if your father has any reversible cause for his confusion or any treatable medical conditions that may have caused the fall. An opinion is needed from a specialist in the medical care or mental health of older people (a geriatrician or old age psychiatrist). Any improvement in mental function will help your father to cooperate better with physiotherapy, thereby ensuring that his potential for rehabilitation has been properly explored and that the therapists have not given up too soon.

Confusion and immobility are common reasons for needing care in a nursing home. The level of dependency and ongoing need should be assessed by the nursing staff and a social worker if local authority funding is needed (a community care assessment). The assessment should be shared with your father or his next of kin. Health and social services provide three types of continuing care:

- continuing social care, which includes home care or residential care;

- continuing health and social care, for example nursing care and personal or social care in a nursing home. The NHS pays the nursing home for the nursing care under a system called the Registered Nurse Care Contribution ('free nursing care'). Payments depend on the level of need arranged in three bands. Both types of continuing care are subject to means testing;

- continuing NHS health care, which is entirely free of charge. Access to this is governed by eligibility criteria contained in a *Joint Policy on Continuing Health and Social Care*, published by each Strategic Health Authority in partnership with its Local Authority. These criteria usually emphasize the degree of dependency, medical instability and frequent need for nursing and medical intervention, so few people qualify. The NHS usually funds this in a dedicated hospital ward or a nursing home, and rarely in a person's own home. Hospital staff considering nursing home care for your father should initially assess whether or not he is eligible for continuing NHS health care.

In order to achieve a satisfactory and fair solution, it is essential that there should be good communication between your father, yourself and all the professionals involved. If, in the end, you are still unhappy with the proposed options, you can appeal against the decision, or you can make a complaint to the ward or the hospital. If you need help in making an appeal or a complaint, you should approach the Patient Advice and Liaison Services (PALS) Officer at the hospital. (See Chapter 4 for more information on PALS and what they do.)

If you agree on nursing home placement you should help choose two or three for which your father would wait if there are no vacancies. Many patients do wait in hospital but health bodies are increasingly considering the option of transferring those who are waiting to other nursing homes, which are not the preferred choice of the individual.

14
Research and clinical trials

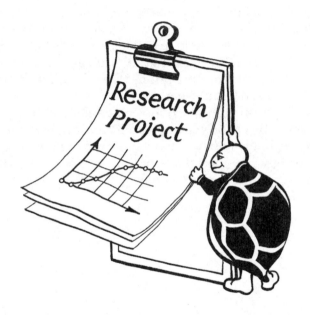

Research – the careful and systematic search for answers – is very important for conditions such as Parkinson's for which there is currently no cure. Research is also important when (again as in Parkinson's) there are various treatments available, none of which is perfect.

In this chapter we consider three different aspects of research: medical research; the clinical trials which are a common feature of such research; and other research projects in related fields which can throw light on the management of Parkinson's, the delivery of services, and the overall quality of life of people with Parkinson's. Our aim is to give an overview of the state of research at the time this book was written. We do not claim that our answers are comprehensive, as new discoveries are taking place all the time and it is impossible to be completely up to date.

Research in Parkinson's disease is funded by a number of sources, including the Medical Research Council, the NHS and the Wellcome Trust. Drug companies' and other industrial research and development programmes for new treatments are also expanding.

The PDS funds a considerable amount of Parkinson's research in the UK, under the auspices of their Research Advisory Panel. This includes an internationally renowned Parkinson's Brain Tissue Bank in London. Further information on the research programme can be obtained from the PDS Research Department. There is also a booklet, called *Seeking Solutions* (B35), which provides details of current PDS funded research. Articles on research are a regular feature of the PDS quarterly magazine, *The Parkinson*, and are being developed on the PDS website. PDS also has SPRING (Special Parkinson's Research Interest Group) for people who wish to keep up with medical research findings. See Appendix 1 for contact details.

Medical research

What progress is being made in identifying the cause of Parkinson's?

Before answering this question, it is worth us spending a little time recapping on the nature of Parkinson's. It is a degenerative disorder which becomes increasingly common with advancing age. The *degeneration of nerve cells* (this is defined in the **Glossary**) found in Parkinson's occurs mainly in one small part of the brain.

This pattern of selective loss of cells is also found in other degenerative conditions, for example in Alzheimer's disease, motor neurone disease and *atypical parkinsonism (Parkinson's Plus syndromes)*. This similarity means that research findings in any one of these conditions may throw light on the causes of the other conditions as well.

One strand of research in Parkinson's is concerned with the scars or marks (called *Lewy bodies*) which are left when nerve cells die. Understanding the proteins which make up these microscopic structures may turn out to be very important. Recently, the protein alpha synuclein has been found in Lewy bodies and researchers are actively investigating how it reacts locally with other proteins in both its normal and abnormal forms, and how, in certain circumstances, such reactions can lead to cell death.

In the last few years more clues to the causes of Parkinson's have been discovered than ever before, thanks – perhaps surprisingly – to some American drug addicts! This modern era of research dates from the early 1980s when a group of young drug addicts in America developed an illness that looked just like Parkinson's. They had taken a drug of abuse containing MPTP. The chemical involved in this drug is a relatively simple one, and it came as a great surprise to researchers to find that such a drug could cause the death of those specific nerve cells that are affected in Parkinson's whilst leaving the rest of the brain and body alone.

Researchers then discovered that MPTP can cause Parkinson's in monkeys so, for the first time, they had an animal model to help test their theories.(We recognize that some people have strongly held views both for and against the use of animals in medical research, but we do not think that a book of this type is the right place to explore such controversies.) MPTP was found to damage particular parts of the cell called the *mitochondria* – the energy pack of the cell. When the mitochondria fail, a number of other biochemical processes also fail and lead to the death of the nerve cell. It was also thought that chemicals like MPTP might produce other compounds called *oxygen free radicals* which are known to have the ability to cause cell damage. Studies done on post-mortem samples of brain from people with Parkinson's have provided evidence that both mitochondrial damage and activation of free radicals do indeed occur. There are also increased iron levels and reduced levels of glutathione, a chemical which helps to protect cells against damage. These are important clues which may lead researchers closer to the cause of Parkinson's.

One possibility is that there are other chemicals, perhaps in the environment or in food, which are rather like MPTP. Some people may have a genetically determined weakness in their defence system against chemicals which means that, unlike unaffected people, they are unable to break them down in their bodies into other harmless substances. The compounds could then cause damage to the substantia nigra (there is a diagram in Chapter 1 showing the position of the substantia nigra).

The availability of an animal model may also help researchers to identify ways in which the damage caused can be halted or even reversed. It has already helped with the development of new dopamine agonists (there is more information about these drugs in Chapter 3) and with the evaluation of *fetal cell implants* and other surgical procedures.

I hear that there has been some progress in understanding the role of genetics in Parkinson's. Is this true?

Yes, the biggest advance since the first edition of this book has been the discovery (in one Italian family where Parkinson's had definitely appeared through several generations) of a defective gene on the fourth chromosome. This gene makes the protein alpha synuclein, now known to be a component of the Lewy body. Even though this is only one, very rare case, it may help researchers to unravel the links between the defective gene, the defective protein which it makes, and the death of dopamine cells. In doing so, it may provide major clues about what goes wrong in more prevalent types of Parkinson's – and how it could be put right.

A second genetic defect which is somewhat more common has been discovered and involves another protein called parkin. This type of Parkinson's is inherited in a different way and does not cause Lewy bodies.

Other genes in other rare families are being discovered (already at least 10 conveniently named PARK genes), and ultimately we will understand these genetic cases and, in turn, those where there is a mixture of genetic and environmental causes.

In order to help future research, people with Parkinson's will increasingly be asked to provide blood samples so that DNA can be extracted. Although it is only in exceptional cases that the information obtained from the DNA will be useful to an individual or family, it can be included in 'group data' for research studies. These may not only be for investigations into the cause of Parkinson's, but also into reasons why different people respond differently to drugs *(pharmocogenetics)*. One common thread in all of the genetic discoveries so far discovered is that the mutant gene causes the abnormal amount or kind of protein produced to interfere with a cellular system known as 'ubiquitination'. This system tags damaged proteins and eliminates them so that they cannot further damage the cell. Although the cause of the initial damage is not understood, ways of improving elimination and therefore reducing accumulation of damaged protein may reduce disease progression.

What other areas of current Parkinson's research seem most encouraging?

Researchers are currently concentrating on four major areas: identifying people at risk; preventing further progression after diagnosis; repairing the damaged brain; and developing new drugs and operations.

Much current research is aimed at trying to find out whether or not we can identify people with Parkinson's before they ever get their first symptom, perhaps by using some form of biochemical test or some sort of scanning device. PET scanning (see the *Glossary* for a definition) can show the loss of the dopamine cells and pathways in Parkinson's, but these machines are very expensive and there are currently only a few in the whole of Britain. A new, but related, type of scanning, SPECT (see the *Glossary* for a definition), may become more widely available over the next few years. It uses a *tracer* (a small dose of a radioactive chemical which is injected into the bloodstream) that can show Parkinson's on the ordinary gamma cameras, available in most hospitals. Knowledge of how cell damage occurs might help us to prevent symptoms emerging in those people shown to be vulnerable, either by improving their defences or by helping them avoid whatever was likely to trigger the appearance of symptoms.

Such understanding of the mechanisms of nerve cell damage may also allow us to prevent further deterioration in people who already have early symptoms. After all, most people are only mildly affected when they are first diagnosed, so if we could just hold it at that point, much would be achieved. Several drugs that may slow down progress are being explored in research trials. Early studies on one called coenzyme Q10 have been published but have been too small to be conclusive. More studies are needed, where the drug would be tested to see if it protects or rescues neurons rather than just helping the symptoms. See the PDS information sheet *Coenzyme Q10* (FS74) for more information.

Methods of repairing brains already seriously damaged by Parkinson's are another avenue for research. The most publicized procedure is that using fetal brain cells but there are other, more distant possibilities. These include the use of other types of cells which have been genetically engineered to contain dopamine, or the identification of substances known as *growth factors* (see the **Glossary** for a definition), which could help the brain to repair itself. Some of these growth factors are already being used in drug trials, especially one called glial-derived neurotrophic factor (GDNF), by direct transfusion into the brain. The results look promising but are not yet conclusive. See the PDS information sheet *GDNF Surgical Research* (FS68) for more information.

The development of new drugs is a major research area. Researchers are looking for new ways of giving Levodopa supplements and attempting to develop new dopamine agonists that are as powerful as levodopa replacement therapy (there is more information about currently available dopamine agonists in Chapter 3). If such dopamine agonists could be developed, it might be possible to eliminate or prevent the fluctuations in response to drugs which we now sometimes see after people have been on treatment for several years. Operations such as pallidotomy and deep brain stimulation (discussed in the section on *Surgical treatments* in Chapter 3) are also a very active area of research.

I watched a programme on TV about stem cell research implants. How significant is this for someone with Parkinson's?

The UK is a major centre for stem cell research and for once is ahead of the USA, largely because of a more enlightened policy by government, and actively encouraged by PDS, the research community and fundraising bodies such as the Medical Research Council and the Wellcome Trust. Parkinson's is widely considered one of the few conditions where such therapy may be a success. However, we cannot expect rapid progress in this area.

Stem cells are unspecialized cells that can divide to produce copies of themselves and can also produce specialized types of cell. Stem cells are found in many different sites in the developing and adult body and brain. They have the ability to develop in different types of cells (e.g. liver, blood, brain, bone) by a process known as differentiation. They also have the ability to renew themselves for long periods and, because they are so versatile, could potentially be used to repair and renew cells in the body and brain.

Stem cells can be derived from several sources, including the very earliest stages of embryo formation, aborted fetuses, blood cells taken from the umbilical cord at birth, bone marrow and even the adult brain.

The cells derived from the early embryo (known as embryonic stem or ES cells) are of particular interest to researchers because they have the capability to develop into all cell types found in the human body. These are one of the main types of stem cell that Parkinson's research is concentrating on.

The aim of stem cell research in Parkinson's is to find a way of inducing the unspecified stem cells to become dopamine cells. In order to do this, stem cell research needs to determine how stem cells remain unspecialized and discover what conditions cause stem cells to become specialized cells.

These are complicated questions, but if they can be answered, in the future it may be possible to develop a treatment whereby stem cells that have been induced to become dopamine cells could be implanted into the brains of people with Parkinson's to replace the missing dopamine nerve cells.

See the PDS information sheet *Stem Cell Research* (FS78) for more information.

Are brain implants using fetal brain material a type of stem cell research?

No. Brain implants using fetal material and stem cell research are both types of neural replacement therapy but the materials and the techniques used are different.

Brain implants using fetal material involve taking developing cells that are already committed to becoming dopamine cells and do not divide when transplanted, whereas transplants involving stem cells would be expected to contain cells that divide and then decide to become dopamine neurones.

The aim of brain implants using fetal dopamine cells is that these cells will connect with the rest of the cells in the brain and start producing enough dopamine to correct the problems that result from a shortage of this neurotransmitter. The results for this type of neural transplant have been mixed.

I have also heard about the prospect of gene therapy. How does this work?

The usual forms of gene therapy use a modified virus that is engineered to contain a gene of importance, such as ones that produce dopamine, growth factors or other neuroprotectants. Again, trials are in progress as we write, but no preliminary data or rumours are available. These trials include 'prosavin' from Oxford Biomedicine, and, in the USA, another controversial trial delivering a therapeutic gene to the subthalamic nucleus, aiming at inhibiting it by increasing the production of gamma-aminobutyric acid (GABA). Gene therapy in other diseases has had a difficult start, causing leukaemia and organ failure, so is heavily regulated by the Department of Health Advisory Committee (GTAC) on gene therapy. As with stem cell and gene therapy, heightened expectations and media interest obscure their exploratory nature and failures are to be expected.

I have heard that Parkinson's drugs could be given by patches on the skin which deliver several doses before having to be replaced. Such a method could be a boon for rather forgetful older people. How soon might this option become a reality?

Skin patches have, as you probably know, proved useful in the treatment of some other conditions such as angina (which affects the heart). Delivery of Parkinson's drugs using skin patches is already available for some anticholinergic drugs, and has certainly been considered for other drugs, because such a system might address the serious problems created by the levels of dopamine in the blood going up and down too quickly.

Patches for a Parkinson's drug, a type of dopamine agonist, are becoming available within trials as we write. As you suggest, patches could be very helpful for people who are rather forgetful but, more importantly, they may help to reduce the fluctuations in response to medication, which people find so distressing.

Clinical trials

How can I find out what drug trials are taking place and whether I am eligible to participate?

We suggest you find out which doctors in your area are particularly interested in Parkinson's. These doctors (who may be either neurologists or specialists in the care of the elderly) are the ones who are most likely to be involved in carrying out drug trials from time to time. Because all drug trials require their volunteers to return to hospital for quite frequent assessments, it is not sensible to get involved in drug trials outside your own area.

Eligibility to take part will vary from one trial to another depending on the type of drug and the questions that the researchers are trying to answer. For example, some drug trials need volunteers who have not yet started on drug treatment for their Parkinson's. Other trials may be trying out new dopamine agonists (there is more information about dopamine agonists in Chapter 3), and for these the researchers usually need people who have been on levodopa for a number of years and who are beginning to develop fluctuating responses to their present treatment.

As well as these 'trial-specific eligibility criteria', there are some more general exclusion criteria that rule out certain groups of people for their own safety. You will usually find that such excluded groups include women who are likely to become pregnant, people with other serious conditions such as heart disease or dementia, and people who are extremely old.

While we applaud your wish to help with research, we would urge you to remember that taking part in a drug trial is not something which should be undertaken without careful consideration – the next two questions raise some of the points that you should consider before agreeing to take part.

I am very disabled and very frustrated, so I do not see why I should not be allowed to try some of the more experimental drugs. However, it seems that you always have to agree to the fact that you may get the placebo. That is no good to me – I have no time to wait.

Although in general there are many drug trials which use *placebos*, they are in fact rather rare in trials for Parkinson's drugs. Most recent Parkinson's drug trials have compared the new drug being tested with the best of the currently available treatments (such as co-careldopa [Sinemet], co-beneldopa [Madopar] or a dopamine agonist). So in these trials everyone is receiving an active treatment.

However, to complete the picture, we shall explain why placebos are used in some instances. It is important to realize that experimental drugs are unproven. Nobody knows if they are going to work or, if they do work, in whom – or if they will have any unwanted side effects. If it was already known that the drug was effective and safe, it would not be necessary to carry out such trials. As it is difficult for either the volunteer (who badly wants an improved drug) or the investigator (who badly wants this new drug to be successful) to be totally objective, it is often necessary to compare the new drug with a placebo (a tablet which looks the same, is harmless, but has no active ingredients). The experimental drug and the placebo have to be allocated 'blind', which means they are given out in a way which ensures that neither the volunteer (as you note in your question) nor the investigator knows who has had which tablet.

When responses to the drug and the placebo are compared at the end of the trial, it is then possible to judge whether the experimental drug has had any real effect. If it is shown to be effective and to have no significant side effects, then it may well become a drug that is used for treatment. We would therefore like to assure you that if you are asked to take part in a drug trial with a placebo, it is because the researchers truly do not know whether the new drug will help you, will make no difference to you, or will even make you worse.

My husband's neurologist is very involved in research and often asks for volunteers. What questions should we ask to ensure that we make the right decisions for ourselves?

People with Parkinson's may be asked to volunteer for several types of research. At the simplest level, there may be requests for a one-off test such as a blood or urine sample. These involve no risk, major discomfort or inconvenience so, if you are satisfied with the reason given for the request, you should be able to decide quite quickly between yourselves whether or not to take part.

The most likely request for volunteers is for participation in a drug trial. More is involved here and you are very sensible to think about the information you need to help you decide about taking part. First of all you need a proper explanation of the reason for the drug trial, and you should receive this both in a face-to-face discussion with your doctor or the researcher, and also in writing. You should not be asked to make an immediate decision at the end of the discussion but, if you are, you should say that you want more time to consider.

During this discussion you can also raise any questions that you have, both about the drug being tested and about practical matters to do with the trial. We list some of the more obvious questions here, but you will probably want to add others of your own.

- Has the drug been given to people with Parkinson's before? If it has, to how many and with what results? (If the results were encouraging, you are more likely to want to take part in a further test.)

- What, if any, side effects can you expect? Any side effects will probably only be minor, as both the drug company and the research ethics committee that has approved the research will have reassured themselves that no serious side effects are likely. Research ethics committees are groups of healthcare professionals, researchers and lay people who review the proposals of researchers to ensure that they are compatible with the protection of the rights, safety, dignity, and well-being of the potential research participants. Further information on research ethics committees is available from the Central Office for Research Ethics Committees (COREC) (see Appendix 1 for contact details).

- Will taking part in the trial cause you any inconvenience?

- How often will you have to return to hospital for tests?

- Will you receive travel expenses?

- How long will the tests and examinations take each time and what will be involved?

- Will the tests be physical examinations, blood tests, psychological tests or something else entirely?

Armed with this information and the written description of the trial, you should then consider your options for a day or two and, if possible, discuss the issues with someone who is approachable and reasonably knowledgeable. This could be your GP or a research nurse, nurse practitioner or Parkinson's Disease Nurse Specialist at the hospital. You can then go back to your doctor or the researcher with any further questions and your decision. Deciding to take part does not commit you to staying in the trial until it is completed – you have the right to withdraw at any time and for any reason (or even for no reason at all).

Many people get a great deal of satisfaction from taking part in research, and doctors and researchers certainly appreciate the cooperation of people with Parkinson's. However, it is important that people take a thoughtful approach, as you are doing, and that they do not feel pressurized in any way to join in a trial or to stay in it if they wish to withdraw.

What protection do volunteers have against injury or illness resulting from participation in clinical trials?

It is, of course, true that there is a small but significant element of risk in any experimental procedure. However, if no risks were ever taken, we should not be able to make progress in research. The important thing is that the risks should be kept to a minimum (through careful application of agreed procedures by the drug companies, the ethics committees and the researchers) and that, as discussed in the previous question, potential volunteers should have full information about the possible risks. Although there have recently been some examples of trials of surgical experiments (where the risks are somewhat higher), most Parkinson's clinical trials will be drug trials. All participants are closely monitored and the results communicated to other interested parties so, if unexpected and undesirable side effects appear, rapid action can be taken.

Before being included in a clinical trial, you will have to sign a consent form stating that you understand what is involved and agree to take part. If there is anything on the consent form that you do not understand, ask. Do not sign until you do.

You do not mention compensation for distress or suffering arising from unexpected side effects, but to complete the picture, we should mention that there is an agreement covering such rare events between the drug companies and the health authorities.

I have heard about requests for donations to the Brain Bank. What is it and what does a donation involve?

The PDS Brain Tissue Bank is based at Imperial College London, which is renowned for its Parkinson's research with extensive Parkinson's clinics, PET imaging and laboratory-based research. Other brain banks exist, for instance, at the National Hospital, Queen Square, and in Newcastle. They are increasingly being linked with banks of DNA samples allowing research on both the genes and what happens in the brain to occur simultaneously. Ordinary 'high street' banks are places where people deposit their money and where skilled bankers use the accumulated wealth to create yet more wealth. The same sort of principles operate in a *tissue bank*, except that in this case only a promise is required during someone's life. Then at death, when the body may seem useless, it suddenly acquires new value as part of the Brain Tissue Bank's deposits, which can then be used by scientists across the UK and internationally to improve our understanding of Parkinson's.

For the Brain Tissue Bank to succeed, three different groups of people need to be involved:

- people (both those with Parkinson's and others who do not have Parkinson's) who are willing to donate their brains or brains plus other organs, and relatives who are willing to carry out their wishes;

- research scientists who will study the brains and other tissues alongside medical information collected during life;

- consultants, GPs and other health professionals (such as Parkinson's Disease Nurse Specialists) who will discuss the project with interested people and be the links between donors and their relatives, specialists and Brain Tissue Bank staff.

The importance of good links between the groups becomes

especially clear when death occurs because, to be really useful, the relevant tissues have to be removed and processed quickly – within 24 hours of death. If you require more information, contact the PDS Brain Tissue Bank. See Appendix 1 for contact details.

Other areas of research

I have found that the physical therapies (I mean physiotherapy, occupational therapy, and speech and language therapy) make an important contribution to my well-being. Is any research taking place in these areas?

There has been growing interest in research into these therapies in recent years, partly because – helpful as the drugs are – many people with Parkinson's still have some problems even when they are on the best possible drug treatment. There are many active researchers investigating management and rehabilitation aspects of Parkinson's involving these therapies, and some of these projects have been funded by the PDS. A big problem in planning research into these therapies is that *double-blind trials* (see the *Glossary* for a definition of these) are not possible, as you cannot pretend to give someone physiotherapy or speech exercises! It is also difficult to gather together large groups of people whose medication will remain unchanged during the time it takes to complete the research.

In spite of these problems some interesting studies have been done to identify particular methods of treatment for problems such as small steps, hurrying gait, freezing in doorways, speech problems and facial immobility.

Another strand of research has looked at the availability of these services, and has found evidence both of lack of referrals to therapists and of shortage of resources. These studies, and the pressure from people with Parkinson's and their relatives, have almost certainly helped to increase awareness of the contribution made by these therapies. There are now more therapists around the country with a special interest in Parkinson's, a development which has been encouraged in the past few years by the development of PDS-funded and managed working parties in physiotherapy, occupational therapy, and speech and language therapy. There is also a network of physiotherapists called the Association of Physiotherapists in Parkinson's Disease Europe (APPDE), which promotes best practice, educational initiatives, and a forum for discussion. Apart from physiotherapists, members also include other professionals, people with Parkinson's and carers. See Appendix 1 for contact details.

Other studies have looked at the best ways of delivering these services (for example, at home rather than in hospitals), and at ways of involving carers and so improving the likelihood that exercises will be continued and good habits maintained when the visits to the therapist come to an end.

Interdisciplinary approaches, where several different professions work together to resolve management of Parkinson's or quality of life issues are also important features of research of this kind.

Have there been any studies about the overall management of Parkinson's?

Yes, there have been a good many. This has been a strand of research very much promoted by the PDS for many years. The PDS has funded several studies looking at the needs of people with Parkinson's and their families, which have helped to identify areas of unmet need, such as information, therapy, care support, transport and social life. Subsequently projects have been developed to try and address areas of concern.

One project attempted to set up a model of good practice which would provide continuity of care, information and multidisciplinary support, including careful consideration of how people are told about their diagnosis. It showed that such team support was acceptable to an unselected group of newly diagnosed people, that it responded to real needs in a flexible way and created a satisfying, viable way for staff to work together. This project, like a later one which concentrated on providing support and counselling around the time of diagnosis, catered for both people with Parkinson's and those with other long-term neurological conditions. A study that focused on communication between doctors and patients illustrated their differing attitudes to the diagnosis of Parkinson's and provided clues about how communication might be made more effective.

Other studies have looked at the needs of people with Parkinson's living in the community, particularly those most seriously disabled, and at ways in which their needs could be met. One study explored the concept of 'quality of life' and found some differences between people with Parkinson's and therapists. Another looked at how care in the community was working out for people with Parkinson's, and found some serious gaps in the 'seamless care' that it had been intended to provide.

All these studies underline the need to listen to people with Parkinson's and to respond in ways appropriate to their individual needs.

Has there been any research addressed to the needs of people who care for those with Parkinson's?

The PDS is committed to funding research relating to carers needs as well as those of people with Parkinson's. All the studies mentioned in the answer to the previous question included attention to the needs of carers. Other studies have had this as their main focus. An early study investigated the causes of stress in carers, and found that the main cause of stress was the occurrence of depression in the person with Parkinson's. This finding directed attention to the need for early diagnosis and treatment of depressive episodes. Another study looked at the effects of caring on the social, psychological and physical well being of carer spouses, and found poorer outcomes for those providing a lot of care. The PDS has also funded research into the impact of falls from the carer's perspective, quality of life for children who have a parent with Parkinson's (some of whom will be actively caring), and depression in carers.

15
The Parkinson's Disease Society

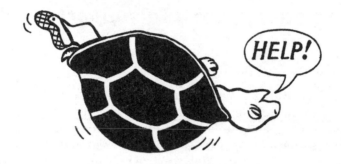

In this book, we have frequently referred to the Parkinson's Disease Society of the UK (PDS for short) – the UK voluntary organization that is dedicated to helping people with Parkinson's and their families. In this chapter we provide information on the Society and the ways in which it supports people with Parkinson's as well as those who care for them. It is a straightforward description of what is available and is not written in question and answer format.

Further information about the PDS, its branches and special interest groups can be obtained by filling in the form at the back of this book or simply by contacting the Society at the address given at the end of this chapter.

Aims

The PDS was founded in 1969 by a very determined and charismatic lady called Miss Mali Jenkins, who had just retired when one of her sisters, Sarah, was diagnosed with Parkinson's. Finding that there was no organization to offer them support, they decided to start one with the help of relatives and friends. In the beginning the main aim was to provide information and help to people with Parkinson's and their families. However, as the PDS has grown, the range of services it provides has expanded.

Information, care and support services

Information and publications

The PDS produces a wide range of publications, information sheets and audiovisual materials on Parkinson's and related subjects. A complete publications list is available on request from the PDS (see Appendix 1 for details). The list can also be viewed and many publications downloaded from the PDS website (www.parkinsons.org.uk).

The Society also has a quarterly membership magazine, *The Parkinson*, which provides up-to-date information on new developments in Parkinson's research, welfare and information. It also provides a forum for people affected by Parkinson's to exchange experiences, hints and tips, etc.

The PDS also deals with individual enquiries on a wide range of aspects of Parkinson's, not covered in the publications. If necessary, it can also refer people to another organization or agency that can provide the information needed.

Helpline

The PDS has a confidential Helpline (available Mondays to Fridays between 9.30 am and 5.30 pm), which offers a listening ear to help anyone with Parkinson's or carers who want to discuss Parkinson's and its treatment, or talk about how they feel. The number is 0808 800 0303 or textphone (Minicom) 020 7963 9380.

Regional and local support

In addition to the national information and support services described above, the PDS has staff working locally across 14 areas in the UK, including Scotland, Northern Ireland and Wales. They aim to ensure that people with Parkinson's and their families have better access to and improved quality of services locally. The activities that they are involved in include local branch support (see below), development of Parkinson's Disease Nurse Specialists and other local services, and building partnerships between lay and professional people.

The PDS has over 300 branches and support groups across the UK. Each branch will be different but in general they all offer opportunities for self-help, mutual support, emotional and practical help, social and educational activities, and fundraising. They generally also have a good knowledge of other local organizations in their particular area that can provide further help and advice on a whole variety of topics. Many also have community support workers who can visit people in their homes to provide information on Parkinson's and local services.

Although all branches arrange regular opportunities for members to meet each other to exchange information and for recreation, it is important to understand that such meetings are only a part of branch activities, and that there is no obligation to attend them. Most branches try to respond to enquirers in whatever way is best suited to their individual needs and wishes, so it is perfectly possible to ask for written information, to exchange ideas or to ask questions over the phone rather than attending the meetings.

As branches are mutual help organizations, many people join in the hope of serving others as well as helping themselves. In addition to being involved with the running and organization of the group, branch members may also take an active part with members of other voluntary groups in making the voice of the users/consumers of health and social services heard in local forums to influence decisions made about these issues. If you are interested in volunteering, there will be no shortage of things for you to do!

For information on your local branch, see the PDS website or contact the Branches Support Unit at the PDS London office.

Younger people with Parkinson's and their families

Although Parkinson's is more common in older people, it is estimated that about 1 in 20 of people diagnosed will be aged under 40 years. The PDS has an information pack for younger people with Parkinson's called *One in Twenty* (B77). This contains information on issues affecting people with young-onset Parkinson's and contributions for younger people with Parkinson's on how they cope.

There is also a special interest group for younger people (i.e. those of working age) people and their families called YAPP&Rs (pronounced Yappers – the letters stand for Young Alert Parkinsonians, Partners & Relatives). Since its beginnings in the late 1980s, its membership and influence has grown steadily. Not only is it a very important source of support and encouragement for its members, it is also a source of ideas and energy for the Society as a whole, and many of its members are active in local branches.

The group produces its own lively quarterly magazine called *Yapmag* and has regional subgroups, which arrange informal meetings. National weekend meetings with invited speakers are arranged every 2 years.

Black and minority ethnic communities

Some of the PDS's most important publications are also translated into key minority ethnic languages including Bengali, Cantonese, Gujerati, Hindi, Punjabi, Urdu and Welsh.

Since 1992, the PDS has also had an Outreach Service for black and minority ethnic communities as a result of concern that people affected by Parkinson's from these communities do not appear to have the access to information and practical support that is available in the wider community. As well as people with Parkinson's, the Outreach Service also provides information and support to people from the minority ethnic communities who have, or care for someone with, motor neurone disease, Huntington's disease, Alzheimer's disease, multiple sclerosis and stroke. For further information, contact the Community Services Department at the PDS London office.

Support for relatives and friends (carers)

The PDS recognizes that living with Parkinson's affects relatives and friends as well as the person with the condition. The PDS offers information and support to help carers cope with the practical and emotional aspects of caring. This includes a *Carers Guide* (B71), two videos for carers – *No More Secrets* (V7) which is aimed at new carers, and *The Long-Term Parkinson's Carers Companion – An A-Z Guide* (V9) aimed at those who have been caring for someone with Parkinson's for several years – plus information for children and young people who have a relative with Parkinson's.

Public relations, policy and campaigning

The PDS is recognized as the national voice for people with Parkinson's and their carers. Using the media, advertising and information materials, the PDS, through its public relations programme, aims to raise awareness of Parkinson's amongst the general public, and encourage greater understanding of the problems it can cause. This includes holding a dedicated Parkinson's Awareness Week every year in April.

The PDS also aims to influence government policy and to campaign on issues relating to Parkinson's to ensure the best quality of services. Initiatives include targeting all levels of government on specific issues, working with other organizations to promote common concerns, and participating in any major health or social care developments affecting people with Parkinson's or their families.

Research

The PDS spends over £2 million a year on more than 65 UK-based research projects. Medical research aims to find the cause, cure and prevention of Parkinson's as well as develop new treatments. Health and social care research concentrates on quality of life, rehabilitation and care issues.

In addition to the £2 million plus spent on these research projects, the PDS also funds an internationally acclaimed Brain Tissue Bank in London, which uses donor tissue from people with and without Parkinson's to research the processes in the brain related to parkinsonism.

The PDS also has a special interest group for people interested in medical research called SPRING (Special Parkinson's Research Interest Group). Their activities include increasing the profile of medical research and raising funds to support projects throughout the UK.

Education

The PDS offers a wide range of education initiatives across the UK to promote awareness and understanding of Parkinson's amongst the many health and social care professionals involved in the care of people with Parkinson's. These include information resources, study days, conferences, and a certificate scheme for care staff.

Fundraising

The PDS is almost entirely funded by voluntary donations. Fundraising events and activities are held throughout the UK to raise money to fund the work of the PDS. These include an annual prize draw, Christmas catalogue and product sales, applications for grants to trusts and corporate companies, legacies, and sponsorship events such as the London Marathon and the Great North Run. If you are interested in fundraising there are many ways you could help. Contact the PDS fundraising department for more information or visit the PDS website.

Contacting the PDS/becoming a Member

If you would like further information or support, please don't hesitate to contact the PDS. You do not have to be a member of the PDS to receive help but membership will ensure that you receive the most up-to-date information through our quarterly magazine, *The Parkinson*. Annual membership costs £4.00 (UK residents), £15 (International).

Most PDS publications mentioned in this book can be downloaded free of charge from the PDS website. Paper copies are also available, though postage and packing is charged on all items. Charges are listed on the PDS publications lists.

The PDS can be contacted at:

**Parkinson's Disease Society
of the United Kingdom**
215 Vauxhall Bridge Road
London SW1V 1EJ
Tel: 020 7931 8080
Fax: 020 7233 9908
Helpline (free number): 0808 800 0303
Textphone (Minicom): 020 7963 9380
    (open Monday–Friday, 9.30am–5.30pm)
E-mail: enquiries@parkinsons.org.uk
Website: www.parkinsons.org.uk

YAPP&RS can be contacted via the PDS Helpline or visit their
    website: www.youngonset-parkinsons.org.uk

SPRING can be contacted on 01403 823947 or visit their website:
    http://spring.parkinsons.org.uk

Glossary

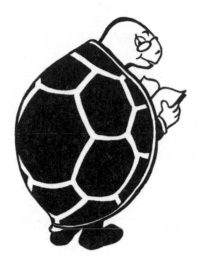

Terms in *italics* in these definitions refer to other terms in the glossary.

acetylcholine A chemical messenger found in the body that transmits
messages between nerve cells or between nerve cells and muscles.
These messages can affect the way muscles behave, or the amount
of saliva produced. Because the actions of acetylcholine are called
cholinergic actions, the drugs that block these actions are called
anticholinergic drugs.

advocate A person who intercedes on behalf of another; someone who
helps vulnerable or distressed people to make their voices heard.

agonists A term used for drugs which have a positive stimulating
effect on particular cells in the body.

Alzheimer's disease The most common type of dementia.

anecdotal evidence Evidence based on the reported experiences of people, rather than scientific evidence such as clinical trials.

anticholinergics A group of drugs used to treat Parkinson's, which work by reducing the amount of acetylcholine in the body, and so facilitate the function of dopamine cells. Drugs in this group are not now used as often as they were before the discovery of *levodopa*.

antidepressants Drugs given to treat depression.

apomorphine A *dopamine agonist* drug which is usually given by injection.

aromatherapy A *complementary therapy* involving treatment with essential oils – often involving massage, but the oils can also be inhaled or added to baths.

atypical parkinsonism The name given to a group of rarer conditions which have some of the symptoms seen in *idiopathic Parkinson's disease* but which progress in unusual or atypical ways. The most common are *multiple system atrophy (MSA)* and *progressive supranuclear palsy (PSP)*.

benign essential tremor Another name for essential tremor.

bradykinesia Slowness of movement.

carbohydrate A class of food which consists of starchy and sugary foods – examples include rice, bread, pasta, potatoes and dried beans.

cardiologist A doctor who specializes in the care and treatment of heart conditions.

care manager A person from a *social services department* or *Primary Care Trust* who is given the task of putting together, monitoring and reviewing the plan of care agreed after a *community care assessment*.

carer In the broadest sense, a carer is anyone who provides help and support of any kind to a relative or friend. More specifically, a carer is a person who is regularly looking after someone who needs help with daily living (perhaps because of age or long-term illness) and who would not be able to live independently at home without this care and support.

carer's assessment An assessment, led by a professional from a *social services* or *social work department*, in which the needs of the carer of someone with a *community care assessment* are considered.

choreiform movements Another name for *involuntary movements*.

clinical trials Closely-supervised scientific studies into treatments for diseases. A clinical trial may investigate a new treatment for a disease, or a different way of giving an existing treatment, or may compare a new treatment with the best treatment currently available.

communication aid Equipment which helps someone who has difficulty with speaking and/or writing to communicate more easily. Communication aids can vary from the very simple, such as alphabet boards or cards with messages already written on them, to the very complex, such as computers.

community care The provision of professional care and support to allow people who need help with daily living (perhaps because of age or long-term illness) to live as full and independent lives as possible (often in their own homes). The amount of care provided will depend on the needs and wishes of the person concerned (which must be taken into account) and on the resources which are available locally.

community care assessment The way in which professional staff from a social services department work out which *community care* services someone needs. The views of the person concerned and of their carers must be taken into account in making the assessment.

complementary therapies Non-conventional health treatments which may be used in addition to conventional medical treatments, such as acupuncture, aromatherapy, reflexology and homeopathy. Some of these therapies are available through the NHS, but this is unusual, and depends on individual hospitals and GPs.

continuous care beds Beds, usually within hospitals but sometimes in *nursing homes*, which are funded by the NHS for people who need permanent medical care.

controlled release Special formulations of drugs that release the drug into the body slowly and steadily rather than all at once. They keep the amount of drug in the blood stream at a steadier level than the 'ordinary' version of the same drug.

corticobasal degeneration An extremely rare kind of *atypical parkinsonism* characterized by jerky movements and a hand or arm that is very clumsy and out of control.

counselling Counsellors are trained to listen carefully to what someone is saying about a particular problem or experience, and then to respond in a way which helps that person to explore and understand more clearly what they are thinking and feeling about that situation. Counselling therefore provides an opportunity for talking openly and fully about feelings without the worry of upsetting close friends or family members. It is always private and confidential.

CT scan An x-ray technique which helps doctors to diagnose disease. The x-rays are passed through the body from many different directions, and are then analysed by a computer to produce cross-sectional pictures of the body.

deep brain stimulation A surgical procedure used to treat Parkinson's involving the implanting of a wire in carefully chosen parts of the brain, such as the pallidum or *subthalamus*, and connection to an apparatus rather like a pacemaker which is implanted in the wall of the chest. This apparatus, which can be switched on and off with a magnet, can send electrical signals to stimulate the chosen part of the brain. It is being used to treat some people with very severe Parkinson's symptoms that are not responsive to drug treatment.

degeneration of nerve cells Death of nerve cells which cannot be explained by infection, blockage of blood vessels or failure of the immune system. Such degeneration is part of the ageing process but in conditions such as Parkinson's, it happens more rapidly than normal.

dementia A disorder in which certain brain cells die more quickly than in normal ageing. The main symptoms are loss of memory and loss of the ability to do quite simple everyday tasks.

depression Feeling sad, hopeless, pessimistic, withdrawn and generally lacking interest in life. Most people feel depressed at some points in their lives, usually in reaction to a specific event such as a bereavement. Doctors become concerned when these feelings persist, especially when there was no obvious outside cause to trigger the feelings in the first place. The physical signs of depression include coping badly, losing weight and not responding well to medication: doctors may diagnose depression from these signs even in someone who claims not to feel depressed.

dietitian A health professional trained in nutrition who can provide advice and information on all aspects of diet and eating behaviour.

DNA (deoxyribonucleic acid) Molecules in cells, which carry genetic information.

dopa-agonists Another name for *dopamine agonists*.

dopa-decarboxylase inhibitors Dopa-decarboxylase is a substance made in the body which converts *levodopa* into *dopamine*. Dopa-decarboxylase inhibitors are drugs which stop this substance working until the *levodopa* in the blood stream reaches the brain. This prevents the side effects which can occur if levodopa is taken on its own.

dopamine A chemical messenger produced by cells in a part of the brain called the *substantia nigra*. Its function is to pass messages from the brain to other parts of the body, particularly to those parts involved in the coordination of movement. Dopamine is in short supply in people who have Parkinson's.

dopamine agonists A group of drugs used to treat Parkinson's. They work by stimulating the parts of the brain which use *dopamine*.

dopamine replacement therapy Treatment with drugs co-beneldopa (Madopar) and co-careldopa (Sinemet), which contain levodopa. When the levodopa reaches the brain it is converted into dopamine, making up for the short supply of this chemical messenger in people with Parkinson's.

double-blind trials A type of *clinical trial* often used in testing the effectiveness of drugs and medicines. It ensures that neither the researcher nor the person taking part in the trial knows whether the drug being given in any individual case is the active medicine or a *placebo*. The aim of this type of trial is to make the research as objective as possible.

dribbling Another word for *drooling*.

driving assessment A test, which takes place at a specially staffed and equipped centre, of someone's ability and fitness to drive a car (with or without special adaptations).

drooling Having saliva overflowing from the mouth.

drug-induced Parkinson's Parkinson's-type symptoms caused by taking certain types of drugs, usually those used for severe psychiatric problems or dizziness. The symptoms can wear off with time when the drugs are stopped.

drug trials A name for *clinical trials* in which drugs are the treatments which are being tested.

dyskinesias Another name for *involuntary movements*.

dystonia An involuntary contraction of the muscles which causes the affected part of the body to go into a spasm (i.e. to twist or tighten).

Such spasms can be painful and can produce abnormal movements, postures, or positions of the affected parts of the body.

encephalitis lethargica Encephalitis means inflammation of the brain and this particular type, which is caused by a virus, makes people very slow and tired (lethargic). It is rarely, if ever, seen now, but there was an epidemic of it after World War I. It often led to a particular type of Parkinson's called 'post-encephalitic Parkinson's'.

epidemiology A branch of medical research which tries to establish the frequency with which diseases occur. For example, it might be used to try to find out how many people in a population of 100,000 have Parkinson's, how many of these people are male and how many female, and how the people with Parkinson's are distributed among different age groups.

erectile dysfunction The preferred term for *impotence*.

essential oils Aromatic (scented) oils extracted from the roots, flowers or leaves of plants by distillation. The complex chemicals in the oils can affect the nervous and circulatory systems of the body and so are considered to have therapeutic properties.

essential tremor A type of *tremor* which often runs in families and which is different from the tremor found in Parkinson's. Essential tremor is at its worst with the arms outstretched or when holding a cup of tea or writing, whereas the tremor of Parkinson's is usually most obvious when the arm is doing nothing and at rest.

familial tremor Another name for *essential tremor*.

fetal cell implants A experimental surgical technique involving implanting cells from aborted fetuses (unborn babies) into the brain of someone with Parkinson's in the hope of repairing the damage that the Parkinson's has caused.

free radicals Highly active chemical units which can be produced by the body or absorbed from outside sources (such as cigarette smoke or polluted air). They only last for very short periods of time, but have the potential to do damage to the body's cells during that time. The body has defence mechanisms against free radicals, but if it is unable to dispose of them fast enough, then cell damage results.

freezing The symptom, quite common in Parkinson's, which causes the person affected to stop suddenly while walking and to be unable to move forward for several seconds or minutes. It makes people feel that their feet are frozen to the ground.

genes The 'units' of heredity that determine our inherited characteristics, such as eye colour.

geriatrician A doctor who specializes in the care and treatment of elderly people.

glaucoma A disease affecting the eyes, usually found in older people. In glaucoma, the pressure of the fluid in the eye becomes so high that it causes damage, and the field of vision becomes progressively narrower and shallower. If left untreated, it can lead to blindness.

glial-derived neurotrophic factor (GDNF) A nerve growth factor, taken from glial cells. It helps develop and control a number of different types of nerve cells, including those that produce dopamine. Used in gene therapy and in a new surgical technique involving the infusion of chemicals in the basal ganglia.

growth factors Natural substances produced in the body which help cells to grow in embryos and foetuses (unborn babies) and which also help adult cells to remain healthy. It is hoped that research into growth factors and the way they work may lead eventually to discovering ways of using these substances to help damaged cells in the brain and central nervous system to regenerate (repair themselves and grow again). Conditions such as Parkinson's which affect the brain and central nervous system are difficult to treat because cells in these parts of the body have very limited capacities for repair and regrowth. It might be possible in the future to use growth factors to make these cells behave more like cells in some other parts of the body (e.g. the skin) which already have the ability to regenerate.

home care worker Usually a person who provides help with personal care, such as getting washed and dressed, and with preparing meals. Home care workers are normally provided by *social services departments*, and there is usually a charge for their services.

home help Usually a person who provides help with shopping, cleaning and similar household tasks but who does not usually provide personal care. Home helps are normally provided by *social services departments*, and there is usually a charge for their services.

homeopathy A *complementary therapy* based on the principle that 'like can be cured by like' (the word homeopathy comes from two Greek words that mean 'similar' and 'suffering'). The remedies used (which are completely safe) contain very dilute amounts of a substance which in larger quantities would produce similar symptoms to the illness being treated. Although there is as yet no scientific explanation for why homeopathy works, it is available through the NHS, although the provision is limited.

idiopathic A word used before the name of an illness or medical condition which means that its cause is not known.

impotence Failure of erection of the penis.

inhibitors A term used for drugs which have a blocking effect on particular cells or chemical reactions in the body.

involuntary movements Movements, other than *tremor*, which are not willed or intended by the person affected. They tend to occur in people who have had Parkinson's for many years and to be related, often in complex and variable ways, to the timing of medication.

levodopa A substance one step removed from *dopamine*. It is not possible for dopamine to pass from the blood stream to the brain, so the problem is solved by giving drugs containing levodopa. The levodopa can reach the brain from the blood stream, and when it gets there it is converted into dopamine.

levodopa Another name for *L-dopa*.

Lewy bodies Microscopic structures seen in the brains of people with Parkinson's.

Lewy body disease (the preferred term is dementia with Lewy bodies) A neurological condition that has symptoms similar to Parkinson's and Alzheimer's diseases.

mask face Another name for *poker face*.

micrographia The technical name for small handwriting. It comes from two Greek words, 'mikros' meaning little and 'graphein' meaning to write.

mitochondria A part of each cell in the body. It is the 'power pack' of the cell and if it is damaged the cell dies.

monoamine oxidase B A naturally-occurring chemical found in the body which causes the breakdown of *dopamine*.

monoamine oxidase inhibitors (MAOIs) A type of drug which falls into two types: Type A (drugs like isocarboxazid [Marplan]; phenelzine [Nardil]; tranylcypromine [Parnate]), which are used to treat depression and anxiety. Owing to their potential interactions with other drugs, they are not usually suitable for people with

Parkinson's. Type B inhibitors, such as selegiline hydrochloride (Elderpryl or Zelapar), prevent the break down of dopamine and are used to treat Parkinson's.

motor disorders Conditions in which damage or disease to the central nervous system causes difficulties in controlling bodily movements.

MPTP A poisonous chemical contained in some drugs of abuse used by young American drug addicts in the early 1980s. It produced an illness with symptoms very similar to those found in Parkinson's.

MRI scan Newer than CT scanning, MRI uses magnetic charges rather than X-rays to image the brain. It is rarely used in the diagnosis of Parkinson's, because, like the CT scan of those with this condition, it usually looks normal.

multidisciplinary assessment An assessment, involving medical, nursing, therapy and social services personnel, of the medical and social care/support someone needs. It is called multi-disciplinary simply because professionals from several different disciplines or specialities are involved!

multiple system atrophy A form of *atypical parkinsonism*. There are usually prominent problems affecting the autonomic nervous system leading to poor bladder control, low blood pressure and impotence.

music therapy The use, by trained professionals, of music as treatment for certain physical and mental illnesses. The music can be used to improve mobility and speech and to enable people to relax or to express feelings and ideas. Music therapists often work with *physical therapists*.

neuroleptics Drugs used to treat schizophrenia and other psychotic disorders.

neurological conditions Conditions affecting the body's nervous system (i.e. the brain and associated nerves).

neurologist A doctor who specializes in the diagnosis, care and treatment of diseases of the nervous system (i.e. the brain and associated nerves).

nursing homes Care homes which offer continuous 24-hour nursing care.

occupational therapists Trained professionals who use specific, selected tasks and activities to enable people who have difficulty with control and coordination of movement to attain maximum function and independence. They also assess people's homes and places of work and suggest ways of making them safer and more manageable. Occupational therapists advise on special aids and gadgets to help with the practical problems of daily living, and on leisure activities to help improve the quality of daily life.

on/off phenomenon This phenomenon is characteristic of some people with long-standing Parkinson's. It can cause them to change from being 'on' and able to move, to being 'off' and virtually immobile, all within a very brief period of time – minutes or even seconds.

optician (also called dispensing optician) They advise on, fit and supply glasses and, if they have had further specialist training, can also fit contact lenses. They do not prescribe glasses/lenses. This is done by an *optometrist*. In the UK the term optician is often used instead of optometrist, but unless an optician is also a trained optometrist, they do not prescribe glasses/lenses.

optometrist (also known as ophthalmic optician) These are highly trained professionals who examine the eyes, give advice on visual problems, prescribe and fit glasses or contact lenses. They also recommend other treatments or visual aids where appropriate and recognize eye disease, referring such cases as necessary. In the UK all optometrists must be qualified and registered. Look for the letter FCOptom or MCOptom after their name. This means that they are a fellow or member of the College of Optometrists and adhere to high standards of clinical practice.

osteopathy A system of diagnosis and treatment involving manipulation of the bones and muscles, commonly used to treat back and joint pain, joint stiffness and similar conditions.

oxygen free radicals *Free radicals* of oxygen which are toxic unless neutralized quickly.

pallidotomy A type of *stereotactic surgery* used to treat Parkinson's which involves making a lesion in the part of the brain called the globus pallidus.

Parkinson's Disease Nurse Specialist A nurse who specializes in Parkinson's disease, and works closely with people with Parkinson's, carers, doctors and other health professionals.

Parkinson's Plus syndromes Also called *atypical parkinsonism*, these are rare conditions whose early symptoms look like Parkinson's but which later develop in rather different ways.

Patient Advisory and Liaison Services (PALS) All trusts running hospitals, GP practices or community health services have a Patient Advice and Liaison Service (PALS). These are designed to offer on the spot help and information, practical advice and support with the aim of resolving any problems or difficulties that people experience while using any NHS service.

pavement vehicle A motorized wheelchair or scooter suitable for use outdoors.

PET scan A type of scan that can 'show' Parkinson's (see also *SPECT scan*). As yet it is only available in some research centres.

physical therapies A group of therapies which includes *occupational therapy*, *physiotherapy* and *speech and language therapy*.

physiotherapy Physical treatments (including exercises) which are used to prevent or reduce stiffness in joints and to restore muscle strength.

placebo The name given in *double-blind trials* to the non-active substance with which an active drug is being compared. It is a 'dummy' version of the drug, identical in appearance to the drug being tested.

poker face Lack of the facial expressions that indicate emotions, for example frowning and smiling.

Primary Care Trusts (PCTs) The local organizations within the NHS that are responsible for the planning, securing and improvement of local health services. They work to ensure that there are integrated health and social care services, better support to local health services and better access, and that there is community engagement in public health and care initiatives.

progressive supranuclear palsy Also known as *Steele–Richardson–Olszewski disease*, this is a form of *atypical parkinsonism*, characterized by relatively poor response to antiparkinson's drugs, early falls and defective eye movements.

protein A class of food that is necessary for the growth and repair of the body's tissues – examples include fish, meat, eggs and milk.

randomized controlled trial Studies, considered to be the gold standard in research, in which a treatment is compared with one or more alternatives or with a *placebo*. Also equal numbers of participants are allocated to each treatment on an entirely random basis. Where possible these allocations are kept concealed from both participants in the trial and doctors to guard against bias. See *double-blind trial.*

Research ethics committee (REC) A group of healthcare professionals, researchers and lay people who review the proposals of researchers to ensure that they are compatible with the protection of the rights, safety, dignity and well-being of the potential research participants. Local RECs, of which there are around 200 in the UK, each cover an area, such as a Strategic Health Authority in England, Health Boards in Scotland, regions of the NHS Wales Department, and in Northern Ireland the Health and Personal Social Services Department. There are also 13 multicentre RECs which each cover the whole of the UK.

residential homes Accommodation for people who are no longer able or who no longer wish to manage everyday domestic tasks (such as cooking, shopping, housework and so on) or to maintain an independent home of their own, but who do not need nursing care.

respite care Any facility or resource which allows those who care for sick, frail, elderly or disabled relatives or friends to have a break from their caring tasks. Respite care may be provided in residential or nursing homes, in the person's own home, or with another family.

resting tremor A name sometimes used for the type of *tremor* found in Parkinson's.

restless leg syndrome Legs that regularly burn, prickle or ache, especially in bed at night. The cause is not known.

rigidity The name given to the special type of stiffness which is one of the main symptoms of Parkinson's. The muscles tend to pull against each other instead of working smoothly together.

season ticket Shorthand name for a prepayment certificate for NHS prescriptions.

self-referral Going direct to a therapist for treatment rather than through a GP or other health professional.

senile tremor Another name for *essential tremor.*

sheltered housing Accommodation which is purpose-built for people who need a certain amount of supervision because of old age or disability, but who wish to maintain a home of their own. The amount of supervision available can vary from a warden on site who can be contacted in an emergency to high-dependency units where there is still a degree of privacy and independence, but where higher staffing levels allow assistance with meals and personal care.

Shy–Drager syndrome Also known as *multiple system atrophy*, this is a form of *atypical parkinsonism*. Falls and weakness of eye movement are common.

side effects Almost all drugs affect the body in ways beyond their intended therapeutic actions. These unwanted 'extra' effects are called side effects. Side effects vary in their severity from person to person, and often disappear when the body becomes used to a particular drug.

sleeping sickness In this book, another name for *encephalitis lethargica*.

social services departments The departments of local authorities responsible for non-medical welfare care for children and adults who need such help.

social work departments The name used in Scotland for local authority departments responsible for the non-medical welfare care of children and adults who need such help.

SPECT scan A scan that uses a radioactive tracer to visualize the brain. New tracers are currently being developed which will be helpful in diagnosing Parkinson's disease, but the test is not widely available and, in any case, is often unnecessary.

speech and language therapists Trained professionals who help with problems concerning speech, communication or swallowing.

Steele-Richardson Olszewski syndrome Also known as *progressive supranuclear palsy*, this is a form of *atypical parkinsonism*.

stereotactic or stereotaxic surgery A type of brain surgery involving the insertion of delicate instruments through a specially created small hole in the skull, and then the use of these instruments to operate on deep structures in the brain which are concerned with the control of movement. The forms of stereotactic surgery used in Parkinson's are *pallidotomy*, *subthalamotomy* and *thalamotomy*.

striatonigral degeneration Also known as *progressive supranuclear palsy (PSP)* or *Steel–Richardson–Olszewski disease*, this is a form of *atypical parkinsonism*.

subcutaneous Under the skin.

substantia nigra So-called because of its dark colour (the name literally means 'black substance'), this part of the brain coordinates movement and contains cells that make dopamine. It is cells from the substantia nigra which are lost or damaged in Parkinson's.

subthalamotomy A type of *stereotactic surgery* performed on the *subthalamus*.

subthalamus A part of the brain that becomes overactive in Parkinson's disease.

syringe driver A small, battery driven pump which can deliver a continuous dose of medication through a flexible line (fine tube) which ends in a needle which is inserted under the skin. It allows people with serious *on/off* Parkinson's to receive a continuous infusion of *apomorphine* and to top this up with occasional booster doses as necessary.

thalamus A part of the brain (located near the *substantia nigra*) which is responsible for relaying information from the sense organs about what is going on in the body to the various parts of the brain.

thalamotomy A type of *stereotactic surgery* performed on the *thalamus*. It was used quite extensively in the past (before the advent of *levodopa* and *dopamine replacement therapy*) in the treatment of one-sided tremor, but is rarely used nowadays.

tissue bank A collection of body tissues which can be used for research purposes. People interested in supporting a tissue bank sign an agreement during their lifetime; the tissue is then donated to the bank after their death. Tissue banks are very important research resources, and the Parkinson's Disease Society has its own Brain Tissue Bank.

tracer A radioactive chemical injected into the blood stream to allow features, which would otherwise be invisible, to be seen. Tracers are used in *PET* and *SPECT scans*. As with other radioactive substances, they have to be used very sparingly, thus regular or frequent use of such scans is not an option.

tremor Involuntary shaking, trembling or quivering movements of the muscles. It is caused by the muscles alternately contracting and relaxing at a rapid rate.

wearing off phenomenon In this phenomenon, which is characteristic of some people with long-standing Parkinson's, the effectiveness of the drug treatment is substantially reduced so that it 'wears off' some time before the next dose is due.

yo-yoing Another name for the *on/off phenomenon*.

Appendix 1
Useful addresses

AbilityNet
PO Box 94
Warwick CV34 5WS
Helpline: 0800 269545
Tel: 01926 312847
Fax: 01926 407425
Website: www.abilitynet.org.uk
*Advice and support to help make
the benefits of using computers
available to disabled children and
adults. Can arrange assessment
at home or in the work place for
a fee.*

Age Concern Cymru
4th Floor
1 Cathedral Road
Cardiff CF11 9SD
Helpline: 0800 00 99 66
Tel: 029 2037 1566
Fax: 029 2039 9562
Website: www.accymru.org.uk
*Is actively involved in policy
making and raising public
awareness through research.
Supports the development of local
Welsh branches and refers to
local groups.*

Age Concern England
Astral House
1268 London Road
London SW16 4ER
Helpline: 0800 00 99 66
Tel: 020 8765 7200
Fax: 020 8765 7211
Website: www.ace.org.uk
*Researches into the needs of older
people and is involved in policy
making. Publishes many books
and has useful fact sheets on a
wide range of issues from benefits
to care, and provides services
via local branches. Helpline open
7am–7pm every day.*

Age Concern Northern Ireland
3 Lower Crescent
Belfast BT7 1NR
Helpline: 028 9032 5055
Tel: 028 9024 5729
Fax: 028 9023 5497
Website: www.ageconcernni.org
*National headquarters in
Northern Ireland offering
information and advice on a wide
range of subjects of interest to
people aged 50 or over, including
finding and paying for residential
and nursing homes. Refers to
local branches.*

Age Concern Scotland
113 Rose Street
Edinburgh EH2 3DT
Helpline: 0800 00 99 66
Tel: 0131 220 3345
Fax: 0131 220 2779
Website:
www.ageconcernscotland.org.uk
Information sheets and local
support groups offering a variety
of services to the elderly.

Alzheimer Scotland – Action on Dementia
22 Drumsheugh Gardens
Edinburgh EH3 7RN
Helpline: 0808 808 3000
Tel: 0131 243 1453
Fax: 0131 243 1450
Website: www.alzscot.org
Offers information, home support,
day care and counselling. Provides
training for health professionals
and local support groups.

Alzheimer Society of Ireland
43 Northumberland Avenue
Dun Laoghaire
Co Dublin
Helpline: 00 353 1 800 341341
Tel: 00 353 1 284 6616
Fax: 00 353 1 284 6030
Website: www.alzheimer.ie
Offers information and practical
help to people with dementia and
their carers.

Alzheimer Society, Northern Ireland
86 Eglantine Avenue
Belfast BT9 6EU
Helpline: 0845 300 0336
Tel: 02890 664100
Fax: 02890 664440
Website: www.alzheimers.org.uk
Offers information, advice, home
support and day care centres for
people suffering from dementia.
Has local support groups, training
for health professionals and
undertake research.

Alzheimer's Society
Gordon House
10 Greencoat Place
London SW1P 1PH
Helpline: 0845 300 0336
Tel: 020 7306 0606
Fax: 020 7306 0808
Website: www.alzheimers.org.uk
Information and helpline for
carers of people with Alzheimer's
disease. Has local support groups
and funds research. Arranges
training courses for carers and
health professionals.

AREMCO
Grove House
Lenham
Kent ME17 2PX
Tel: 01622 858502
Fax: 01622 850532
Email: aremco@onetel.net.uk
Supplier of a variety of
equipment, aids and tools for
people with disabilities: protective
headgear, bed-leaving alarms and
swivel seats for cars, etc.

Aromatherapy Consortium
PO Box 6522
Desborough
Kettering NN14 2YX
Tel: 0870 774 3477
Fax: 0870 774 3477
Website:
www.aromatherapy-regulation.org.uk
Umbrella body representing
aromatherapy associations that
sets national standards. Can
provide details of local therapists,
training and general information.
Telephone staffed 10am–2pm
Mon–Fri.

Artsline
54 Chalton Street
London NW1 1HS
Tel: 020 7388 2227
Fax: 020 7383 2653
Minicom 020 7388 2227
Website: www.artsline.org.uk
Campaigns on behalf of artists
with disabilities through
legislation and training. Offers
information on arts and
entertainments venues which have
disabled access for people with
disabilities.

Association of Physiotherapists
in Parkinson's Disease Europe
Felicity Handford, Secretary
rue W Coppens 6
1170 Watermael Boisfort
Brussels, Belgium
Tel: 00 322 673 8050
Website: http://appde.unn.ac.uk
Offers assessment, monitoring,
treatment and management,
referral to other professionals and
agencies and ongoing support for
both individuals with Parkinson's
disease and their carers from
diagnosis to the later stages.

Association of Professional
Music Therapists
61 Church Hill Road
East Barnet EN4 8SY
Tel: 020 8440 6226 (Mon, Tues &
Thurs)
Fax: 020 8440 6226
Website: www.apmt.org.uk
Body which sets standards of
training and practice among
professional music therapists.
Can refer to local music
therapists.

BBC Audio Books
St James House
The Square
Lower Bristol Road
Bath BA2 3SB
Tel: 01225 878000
Fax: 01225 448005
Website: www.audiobookcollection.com
Alternative website:
www.largeprintdirect.co.uk
Books in large print and audio
tapes for sale. Mail order only.

Benefits Agency
The address and telephone number
of your local Benefits Agency will
be in the Phone Book and in
Yellow Pages under Social
Services.
Helpline: 0800 88 22 00
Government agency with
information and advice on all
types of benefits. (See also Benefits
Enquiry Line for people with
disabilities.)

Benefits Enquiry Line (BEL)
[for people with disabilities]
Helpline: 0800 88 22 00
Freephone N. Ireland 0800 22 06 74
Minicom 0800 24 33 55
Website: www.dwp.gov.uk
Government agency giving
information and advice on
sickness and disability benefits for
people with disabilities and their
carers.

Britannia Pharmaceuticals Ltd
41–51 Brighton Road
Redhill RH1 6YS
Tel: 01737 773741
Fax: 01737 762672
Website: www.britannia-pharm.co.uk
Additional website:
www.apomorphine.co.uk
Manufacturer of pharmaceuticals
including apomorphine for people
with Parkinson's.

British Association
of Art Therapists
Southampton Place Business
Centre
16–19 Southampton Place
London WC1A 2AJ
Tel: 020 7745 7262
Website: www.baat.org
Professional association
representing art therapists
worldwide. Promotes art therapy
in the UK and maintains a
directory of qualified therapists.

British Association of
Occupational Therapists
106–114 Borough High Street
Southwark
London SE1 1LB
Tel: 020 7357 6480
Fax: 020 7450 2299
Website: www.baot.org.uk
Professional association for
occupational therapists, providing
information to the public.

British Complementary
Medicine Association
PO Box 5122
Bournemouth BH8 OWG
Tel: 0845 345 5977
Fax: 0845 345 5977
Website: www.bcma.co.uk
Multitherapy umbrella body
representing organizations,
clinics, colleges and independent
schools, and acting as the voice
of complementary medicine.

British Red Cross
9 Grosvenor Crescent
London SW1X 7EJ
Tel: 020 7235 5454
Fax: 020 7245 6315
Website: www.redcross.org.uk
Gives skilled and impartial care
to people in need or crisis in their
own homes, the community, at
home and abroad, in peace and
in war. Refers to local branches.

**British Society
for Disability and Oral Health**
Hon. Secretary
Royal Leamington Spa
Rehabilitation Hospital
Heathcote Lane
Leamington Spa CV34 6SR
Tel: 01926 317726
Website: www.bsdh.org.uk
*NHS dental service for people with
disabilities with dental problems.*

British Telecom
BT Correspondence Centre
TVTE
Gateshead NE11 0ZZ
Tel: 150
Website: www.bt.com/disabilityservices
*Offers advice and practical help to
people who have difficulties using
telephone.*

Calvert Trust
Website: www.calvert-trust.org.uk
*Runs holiday centres for people
with disabilities and their
families.*

Care & Repair Cymru
Norbury House
Norbury Road
Cardiff CF5 3AS
Tel: 029 2057 6286
Fax: 029 2057 6283
Website: www.careandrepair.org.uk
*Innovates, develops, promotes and
supports housing policies and
initiatives that enable elderly and
disabled people to live
independently in their own homes
for as long as they wish. Can refer
to local branches.*

Care & Repair England
3rd Floor, Bridgford House
Pavilion Road
West Bridgford
Nottingham NG2 5GJ
Tel: 0115 982 1527
Fax: 0115 982 1529
Website:
www.careandrepair-england.org.uk
*Innovates, develops, promotes and
supports housing policies and
initiatives that enable elderly and
disabled people to live independently in their own homes for as
long as they wish. Telephone
staffed 8.30am–4.30pm
Mon–Thurs.*

Care & Repair Forum Scotland
236 Clyde Street
Glasgow G1 4JH
Tel: 0141 221 9879
Fax: 0141 221 9885
Website: under development
*Innovates, develops, promotes and
supports housing policies and
initiatives that enable elderly and
disabled people to live
independently in their own homes
for as long as they wish. Can refer
to local branches.*

Carers UK
20–25 Glasshouse Yard
London EC1A 4JS
Helpline: 0808 808 7777
Tel: 020 7490 8818
Fax: 020 7490 8824
Website: www.carersonline.org.uk
*Offers information and support to
all people who are unpaid carers,
looking after others with medical
or other problems. Campaigns at
national level on behalf of all
carers.*

**Central Office for Research
Ethics Committee (COREC)**
Room 76, B Block
40 Eastbourne Terrace
London W2 3QR
Tel: 020 7725 3431
Fax: 020 7725 3465
Website: www.corec.org.uk
*Coordinates policies, development
and training of operational
systems for local and multicentre
research ethics committees on
behalf of the NHS in England.*

**Centre for Accessible
Environments**
Nutmeg House
60 Gainsford Street
London SE1 2NY
Tel: 020 7357 8182
Fax: 020 7357 8183
Website: www.cae.org.uk
*Gives advice and training on new-
build and adaptations to homes,
churches, health centres which are
environmentally accessible for
elderly or disabled people.*

Charity Search
25 Portview Road
Avonmouth
Bristol BS11 9LD
Tel: 0117 982 4060
Fax: 0117 982 2846
Website: under development
*Provides information on sources
of charitable funding for older
people. Telephone staffed
9am–3pm Mon–Thurs.*

**Chartered Society of
Physiotherapy**
14 Bedford Row
London WC1R 4ED
Tel: 020 7306 6666
Fax: 020 7306 6611
Website: www.csp.org.uk
*For information about all aspects
of physiotherapy. Offers list of
registered physiotherapists
around the country.*

The Children's Society
Edward Rudolf House
Margery Street
London WC1X 0JL
Helpline: 0845 300 1128
Tel: 020 7841 4400
Website: www.childrenssociety.org.uk
*Campaigns at government level
on behalf of children. Runs local
projects and, where appropriate,
liaises with other agencies.*

The Cinnamon Trust
Foundry House
Foundry Square
Hayle
Cornwall TR27 4HH
Tel: 01736 757 900
Fax: 01736 757 010
Website: www.cinnamon.org.uk
National charity for elderly or
terminally ill people and their
pets. A team of volunteers cares for
pets if owner is taken ill. Has list
of nursing homes, sheltered
housing for the elderly that will
accept residents and their pets.

Citizens Advice (National
Association – NACAB)
Myddleton House
115–123 Pentonville Road
London N1 9LZ
Tel: 020 7833 2181
Fax: 020 7833 4371
Website: www.adviceguide.org.uk
HQ of national charity offering a
wide variety of practical, financial
and legal advice. Network of local
branches throughout the UK listed
in the Phone Book and in Yellow
Pages under Counselling and
Advice. To volunteer please ring
08451 264264.

College of Optometrists
42 Craven Street
London WC2N 5NG
Tel: 020 7839 6000
Fax: 020 7839 6800
Website: www.college-optometrists.org
Professional college for
optometrists.

Complementary Medical
Association
67 Eagle Heights
The Falcons
Bramlands Close
London SW11 2LJ
Helpline: 0845 129 8434
Tel: 01424 438801
Fax: 0845 1298435
Website: www.the-cma.org.uk
A not-for-profit medical body
offering membership to highly
qualified practitioners of
complementary medicine. Has a
database of accredited
practitioners around the UK.

The Continence Foundation
307 Hatton Square
16 Baldwins Gardens
London EC1N 7RJ
Helpline: 0845 345 0165
Tel: 020 7404 6875
Fax: 020 7404 6876
Website:
www.continence-foundation.org.uk
Offers information and support
for people with bladder and/or
bowel problems. Has lists of
regional specialists. Telephone
helpline staffed 9.30am–1pm
Mon–Fri.

Councils for Voluntary Service
237 Pentonville Road
London N1 9NJ
Tel: 020 7278 6601
Fax: 020 7833 0149
Website: www.csv.org.uk
*UK's voluntary and training
organization that places
volunteers aged 16–35 in
community-based settings with
children, care homes, the elderly
and within schools. For local
branches see your telephone
directory.*

Counsel & Care
Lower Ground Floor
Twyman House
16 Bonny Street
London NW1 9PG
Helpline: 0845 300 7585
Tel: 020 7241 8555
Fax: 020 7267 6877
Website: www.counselandcare.org.uk
*Offers information to people over
60 on welfare rights, benefits,
community care, helps with choice
of residential homes, including
inspection and registration of
units. Some grants available.
Helpline staffed 10am–1pm
Mon–Fri.*

Crossroads Caring for Carers
10 Regent Place
Rugby CV21 2PN
Helpline: 0845 450 0350
Helpline (Wales): 02920 222282
Helpline (Scotland): 0141 226 3793
Tel: 01788 573653
Fax: 01788 565498
Website: www.crossroads.org.uk
*Supports and delivers high quality
services for carers and people with
care needs via its local branches.*

Crossroads Scotland
24 George Square
Glasgow G2 1EG
Tel: 0141 226 3793
Fax: 0141 221 7130
Website:
www.crossroads-scotland.co.uk
*Information leaflets on respite
care and support for carers within
own homes, for any age, disability
and sickness. Local branches.*

Department of Health (DoH)
PO Box 777
London SE1 6XH
Helpline: 0800 555777
Tel: 020 7210 4850
Fax: 01623 724 524
Textphone: 020 7210 5025
Website: www.doh.gov.uk
*Produces literature about health
issues, available via helpline.
A more technical site with
National Service Frameworks
available from the internet,
e.g.* www.doh.gov.uk/nsf/

**Department of Work
and Pensions**
Disability Benefit Centre
3 Olympic House
Olympic Way
Wembley HA9 0DL
Helpline: 0800 88 22 00
Tel: 020 8795 8400
Website: www.dwp.gov.uk
*Government information service
offering advice on benefits for
people with disabilities and their
carers.*

Depression Alliance
35 Westminster Bridge Road
London SE1 7JB
Helpline: 0845 123 2320
Tel: 020 7633 0557
Fax: 020 7633 0559
Website: www.depressionalliance.org
Offers support and understanding
to anyone affected by depression
and for relatives who want help.
Has a network of self help groups,
correspondence schemes and a
range of literature; send SAE for
information.

DIAL UK
St Catherine's
Tickhill Road
Balby
Doncaster DN4 8QN
Tel: 01302 310123
Fax: 01302 310404
Website: www.dialuk.org.uk
National organization for the
DIAL network – 150 disability
advice centres run by and for
disabled people. Offers free and
independent advice by phone and
in drop-in centres on all aspects of
disability. Less mobile clients can
be visited in their homes.

Directory of Social Change
24 Stephenson Way
London NW1 2DP
Helpline: 0845 077707
Tel: 020 7391 4800
Fax: 020 7391 4808
Website: www.dsc.org.uk
Advises voluntary and community
groups how to work most effectively
and campaigns on their behalf.

Disabled Person's Railcard
Office
PO Box 1YT
Newcastle-upon-Tyne NE99 1YT
Tel: 0191 269 0304

Disability Alliance
Universal House
88–94 Wentworth Street
London E1 7SA
Helpline: 020 7247 8763
Tel: 020 7247 8776
Fax: 020 7247 8765
Website: www.disabilityalliance.org
Offers information on benefits
*through publications (*Disability
Rights Handbook*), free briefing*
sheets, rights advice line and
training. Campaigns for
improvements to the social
security system.

Disability Benefits Unit
Warbreck House
Warbreck Hill Road
Blackpool FY2 0YE
Helpline: 0845 712 3456
Textphone 0845 722 4433
Website: www.dwp.gov.uk
Government agency specifically for
queries about and applications for
Disability Living Allowance and
Attendance Allowance. Helpline
staffed 7.30am–6.30pm weekdays.

Disability Rights Commission
Freepost MID 02164
Stratford upon Avon CV37 9BR
Tel: 08457 622633
Fax: 08457 778878
Minicom 08457 622644
Website: www.drc-gb.org
*Government-sponsored centre
offering publications and up-to-
date information on the Disability
Discrimination Act. Special team
of advisers can help with problems
of discrimination at work
8am–8pm weekdays.*

Disability Sport England
Unit 4G, N17 Studios
784–788 High Road
Tottenham
London N17 ODA
Tel: 020 8801 4466
Fax: 020 8801 6644
Website: www.disabilitysport.org.uk
*Provides opportunities for people
of all ages with disabilities to take
part in sport. Has regional offices.*

Disabled Drivers Motor Club
Cottingham Way
Thrapston
Northants NN14 4PL
Tel: 01832 734724
Fax: 01832 733816
Website: www.ddmc.org.uk
*Offers information service to
disabled drivers about ferries,
airports and insurance. Subscrip-
tion for monthly magazine.*

Disabled Living Centres Council
Redbank House
4 St Chad's Street
Cheetham
Manchester M8 8QA
Tel: 0161 834 1044
Fax: 0161 839 0802
Textphone 0161 839 0885
Website: www.dlcc.org.uk
*Coordinates work of Disabled
Living Centres in UK. Offers lists
of centres where you can see
furniture, aids and equipment for
elderly and disabled people. Offers
training courses for professionals.*

Disabled Living Foundation
380–384 Harrow Road
London W9 2HU
Helpline: 0845 130 9177
Tel: 020 7289 6111
Fax: 020 7266 2922
Textphone (Minicom)
020 7432 8009
Website: www.dlf.org.uk
*Provides information to disabled
and older people on all kinds of
equipment in order to promote
their independence and quality of
life. Helpline staffed 10am–1pm
Mon–Fri.*

Driver and Vehicle Licensing Authority (DVLA)
Medical Branch
Longview Road
Morriston
Swansea SA99 1TU
Helpline: 0870 600 0301
Tel: 0870 240 0009
Fax: 01792 761100
Website: www.dvla.gov.uk
Information and advice for motorists with disabilities.

Gardening for the Disabled Trust
c/o F Seton
The Freight
Cranbrook TN17 3PG
Tel: 01580 712196
Volunteers offers practical advice and information to help keen gardeners keep gardening, despite disability or age. Also offers small grants.

General Osteopathic Council
Osteopathy House
176 Tower Bridge Road
London SE1 3LU
Tel: 020 7357 6655
Fax: 020 7357 0011
Website: www.osteopathy.org.uk
Regulatory body that offers information to the public and lists of accredited osteopaths.

Health Development Agency
Holborn Gate
330 High Holborn
London WC1V 7BA
Helpline: 0870 121 4194
Tel: 020 7430 0850
Fax: 020 7061 3390
Website: www.hda-online.org.uk
Formerly Health Education Authority; now only deals with research. Publications on health matters can be ordered on 0800 55 57 77.

Help the Aged
207–221 Pentonville Road
London N1 9UZ
Helpline: 0808 800 6565
Tel: 020 7278 1114
Fax: 020 7278 1116
Website: www.helptheaged.org.uk
Offers advice and a range of free information leaflets on benefits, community and residential care and housing options.

Holiday Care
7th Floor, Sunley House
4 Bedford Park
Croydon CR0 2AP
Helpline: 0845 124 9971
Tel: 0845 124 9974
Fax: 0845 124 9972
Minicom: 0845 124 9976
Website: www.holidaycare.org
Provides holiday advice on venues and tour operators in the UK and abroad for people with special needs. Publishes information sheets on overseas destinations. Offers professional consultancy service to the tourism industry.

Incontact
– Action on Incontinence
United House
North Road
London N7 9DP
Tel: 0870 770 3246
Fax: 0870 770 3249
Website: www.incontact.org
Information and help via local
support and user groups for people
with bladder and bowel problems.
Raises awareness to break the
stigma that still surrounds
incontinence.

Inland Revenue
Website: www.inlandrevenue.gov.uk
Look at local directory for the
appropriate telephone number in
your area.

Institute for Complementary
Medicine
PO Box 194
London SE16 7QZ
Tel: 020 7237 5165
Fax: 020 7237 5175
Website: www.icmedicine.co.uk
Umbrella group for
complementary medicine
organizations. Offers informed,
safe choice to public, British
register of practitioners and refers
to accredited training courses.
SAE requested for information.

J D Williams
(Special Collection)
Griffin House
40 Lever Street
Manchester M60 6ES
Helpline: 0870 160 6100
Tel: 0161 238 2000
Fax: 0161 238 2025
Website: www.jdwilliams.co.uk
A mail order catalogue of fashion
clothing and footwear available in
large sizes.

Jobcentre Plus
Website: www.jobcentreplus.gov.uk
Government centres offering
advice to those seeking, as well as
offering, employment, including
legal issues and benefit claims. See
telephone directory for local
centre.

Keep Able Ltd
Sterling Park
Pedmore Road
Brierley Hill DY5 1TB
Helpline: 0800 169 1609
Tel: 01384 484544
Fax: 01384 480717
Website: www.keepable.co.uk
Distributors of equipment and
aids for the elderly and less able.
Home assessments for stairlifts,
wheelchairs etc. Available via mail
order. Some regional stores.

LearnDirect
Website for information on lifelong learning
Helpline: 0800 10 09 00
Website: www.learndirect.co.uk
University for industry, working with government, BBC Education, Channel 4 and others; offers workforce development and lifelong learning through a network of learning centres 7 days a week 8am–10pm. Courses also available in several Asian languages.

Leonard Cheshire
30 Millbank
London SW1P 4QD
Tel: 020 7802 8200
Fax: 020 7802 8250
Website: www.leonard-cheshire.org
Offers care, support and a wide range of information for disabled people between 18 and 65 years in the UK and worldwide to encourage independent living. Respite and residential homes, holidays and rehabilitation.

Listening Books
12 Lant Street
London SE1 1QH
Tel: 020 7407 9417
Fax: 020 7403 1377
Website: www.listening-books.org.uk
Provide audio books, for both pleasure and learning, on tape for adults and children suitable for anyone who cannot hold a book, turn pages or read in the usual way. Subscription for lending library of tapes by mail order.

Mind (National Association for Mental Health)
Granta House
15–19 Broadway
London E15 4BQ
Helpline: 0845 766 0163
Tel: 020 8519 2122
Fax: 020 8522 1725
Website: www.mind.org.uk
Mental health organization working for a better life for everyone experiencing mental distress. Offers support via local branches. Publications available on 020 8221 9666.

Mobility Advice & Vehicle Information Service (MAVIS)
Department for Transport
Crowthorne Business Estate
Old Wokingham Road
Crowthorne RG45 6XD
Tel: 01344 661000
Fax: 01344 661066
Website: www.mobility-unit.dft.gov.uk
Government department offering driving and vehicle assessment to people with disabilities. Can advise on vehicle adaptations for both drivers and passengers.

Mobility Assessment Centres
see **Mobility Advice and Vehicle Information Service (MAVIS)**
Details of centres are available via MAVIS and in the PDS publication, Parkinson's and Driving *(B64).*

Motability
Goodman House
Station Approach
Harlow CM20 2ET
Helpline: 01279 635666
Tel: 01279 635999
Fax: 01279 632000
Minicom 01279 632273
Website: www.motability.co.uk
*Advises people with disabilities
about powered wheelchairs, scooters,
new and used cars, how to adapt
them to their needs and obtain
funding via the Mobility Scheme.*

National Animal Welfare Trust
Tyler's Way
Watford-By-Pass
Watford WD25 8WT
Tel: 020 8950 0177
Fax: 020 8420 4454
Website: www.nawt.org.uk
*Provides short-term care and
rehabilitation at own rescue
centres for unwanted, ill-treated
and abandoned animals.*

**National Association of
Councils for Voluntary Service**
177 Arundel Street
Sheffield S1 2NU
Tel: 0114 278 6636
Fax: 0114 278 7004
Textphone 0114 278 7025
Website: www.nacvs.org.uk
*Headquarters representing the
growing network of over 300
councils for voluntary service
throughout England. Helps
promote voluntary and
community action at local level.
See local telephone directory for
your nearest branch.*

National Extension College
The Michael Young Centre
Purbeck Road
Cambridge CB2 2HN
Tel: 01223 400 200
Fax: 01233 400 399
Website: www.nec.ac.uk
*Offers a wide range of tailor-made
vocational & professional courses
by distance learning.*

National Gardens Scheme
Hatchlands Park
East Clandon
Guildford GU4 7RT
Tel: 01483 211535
Fax: 01483 211537
Website: www.ngs.org.uk
*Provides list of privately owned
gardens of quality, character and
interest, which, for a donation to
charity, are open to the public at
certain times of year.*

**National Institute for
Conductive Education**
Cannon Hill House
Russell Road
Moseley
Birmingham B13 8RD
Tel: 0121 449 1569
Fax: 0121 449 1611
Website:
www.conductive-education.org.uk
*Charity promoting the use of
conductive education for the benefit
of rehabilitating children and
adults with motor disorders such
as cerebral palsy, Parkinson's,
head injury or stroke.*

National Trust

36 Queen Anne's Gate
London SW1H 9AS
Tel: 0870 609 5380
Fax: 020 7222 5097
Website: www.nationaltrust.org.uk
Promotes the preservation and protection of the coastline, countryside and buildings of England, Wales and N. Ireland. Has many long-term education programmes emphasizing the importance of the environmenmt and preservation of our heritage.

NHS 24 (Scotland)

Helpline: 0800 22 44 88
Website: www.nhs24.com
NHS 24 is the Scottish 24-hour helpline offering confidential healthcare advice, information and referral service 365 days of the year. A good first port of call for any health advice.

NHS Direct (England, Northern Ireland & Wales)

Helpline: 0845 4647
Tel: 020 8867 1367
Textphone: 0845 606 4647
Website: www.nhsdirect.nhs.uk
NHS Direct is a 24-hour helpline offering confidential healthcare advice, information and referral service 365 days of the year. A good first port of call for any health advice.

NHS Health Scotland

Woodburn House
Canaan Lane
Edinburgh EH10 4SG
Tel: 0131 536 5500
Fax: 0131 536 5501
Textphone 0131 536 5503
Website: www.hebs.com
NHS health education board for Scotland publishing leaflets on a variety of health issues.

Open College of the Arts

Registration Department
OCA
Freepost SF10678
Barnsley S75 1BR
Tel: 0800 731 2116
Fax: 01226 730838
Minicom 01226 205255
Website: www.oca-uk.com
A community of artists, writers and designers providing inexpensive arts-based courses to develop creative skills.

Open University (OU)

Office for Students with Disabilities
South West Building
Walton Hall
Milton Keynes MK6 7AA
Tel: 01908 653 745
Fax: 01908 655 447
Website: www.open.ac.uk
Offers advice to people with disabilities who wish to study accredited educational courses at home. Provides materials in alternative format, i.e. tapes, CDs and comb-bound books.

Outsiders
BCM Box Outsiders
London WC1N 3XX
Tel: 020 7354 8291
Website: www.outsiders.org.uk
*Trust campaigns for disabled
people's rights to privacy and a
satisfying personal life. Offers
information via sex and disability
helpline which is staffed by
volunteers on Mondays 1pm–5pm.*

**Parkinson's Association
of Ireland**
Carmichael Centre
North Brunswick Street
Dublin 7
Helpline: 1 800 359 359
Tel: 00 353 1872 2234
Fax: 00 353 18735737
*Offers information, newsletter to
members. Has local support
groups; some exercise classes.*

**Parkinson's Disease
Nurse Association**
Sarah Mason PD Nurse
Belfast City Hospital
91 Lisburn Road
Belfast BT9 7AB
Website: www.pdnsa.org
*Website providing information
and support for nurses caring for
people with Parkinson's disease.*

**Parkinson's Disease Society
(PDS)**
National Office
215 Vauxhall Bridge Road
London SW1V 1EJ
Helpline: 0808 800 0303
Tel: 020 7931 8080
Fax: 020 7233 9908
Minicom 020 7963 9380
Website: www.parkinsons.org.uk
*National UK Parkinson's
organization. See Chapter 15 for
more details of their work.*

**Parkinson's Disease Society
Tissue Bank**
Division of Neuroscience &
Psychological Medicine
Imperial College London
Faculty of Medicine
Charing Cross Campus,
Fulham Palace Road
London W6 8RF
Tel: 020 8383 4917
Fax: 020 8383 4918
Website:
www.parkinsonstissuebank.ic.ac.uk
*Supplies brain and spinal tissue
donated by people with
Parkinson's and control subjects,
to researchers investigating
Parkinson's and related disorders
in the UK and worldwide.*

Patient Advice and Liaison Services (PALS)

Available in all trusts running hospitals, GP practices or community health services. Offer information and support on local NHS services and help to resolve any problems or difficulties that people have using any NHS service. Your GP or Primary Care Trust can provide contact details.

The Patients Association

PO Box 935
Harrow HA1 3YJ

Pet Fostering Service, Scotland

PO Box 6
Callander FK17 8ZU
Tel: 01877 331 496
Website: www.pfss.org.uk
Provides temporary care in an emergency in the homes of volunteer fosterers for the pets of people who cannot make alternative care arrangements. Can refer to local services.

Primary Care Trusts

NHS body that oversees the management of local health services. Telephone number available via your local directory or your GP surgery should be able to advise you.

Princess Royal Trust for Carers

142 Minories
London EC3N 1LB
Tel: 020 7480 7788
Fax: 020 7481 4729
Website: www.carers.org
Offers information on a UK-wide network of independent carer centres, as well as advice and support to all carers. Information available on website or by telephone.

Progressive Supranuclear Palsy (PSP Europe) Association

The Old Rectory
Wappenham
Towcester NN12 8SQ
Tel: 01327 860299
Fax: 01327 861007
Website: www.pspeur.org
Offers information about progressive supranuclear palsy. Has local support groups, and undertakes research worldwide into PSP. Also supports people with corticobasal degeneration.

RADAR (Royal Association for Disability & Rehabilitation)
12 City Forum
250 City Road
London EC1V 8AF
Tel: 020 7250 3222
Fax: 020 7250 0212
Minicom 020 7250 4119
Website: www.radar.org.uk
Campaigns to improve rights and care of disabled people. Offers advice on every aspect of living with a disability and refers to other agencies for training and rehabilitation. Sells special key to access locked disabled toilets.

Rail Unit for Disabled Passengers Switchboard
Helpline: 08700 005151
Rail Information Line:
08457 48 49 50
National call centre dealing with queries about travelling within the UK rail network and referring to appropriate areas for advice. Enquirers must provide specific details of destination in order to be referred to the appropriate railway company.

Relate
Herbert Gray College
Little Church Street
Rugby CV21 3AP
Helpline: 0845 130 4010
Tel: 01788 573241
Fax: 01788 535007
Website: www.relate.org.uk
Offers relationship counselling via local branches. Relate publications on health, sexual, self-esteem, depression, bereavement and re-marriage issues are available from bookshops, libraries or via website. Appointments booking line 0845 130 4016

Research Council for Complementary Medicine
27A Devonshire Street
London W1G 6PN
Tel: 020 7935 7499
Fax: 020 7935 2460
Website: www.rccm.org.uk
Enables research and provides information on existing research. Requests for access to research details can be made via website.

RICABILITY (Research Institute for Consumer Affairs)
30 Angel Gate
City Road
London EC1V 2PT
Tel: 020 7427 2460
Fax: 020 7427 2468
Textphone 020 7427 2469.
Website: www.ricability.org.uk
Researches and publishes consumer guides on products and services which enable older and disabled people to live more easily and independently; SAE requested for publications list.

Royal College of Speech and Language Therapists
2 White Hart Yard
London SE1 1NX
Tel: 020 7378 1200
Fax: 020 7403 7254
Website: www.rcslt.org
Professional association for speech and language therapists, providing information to the public.

Sarah Matheson Trust (multiple system atrophy)
Pickering Unit
St Mary's Hospital
Praed Street
London W2 1NY
Tel: 020 7886 1520
Fax: 020 7886 1540
Website: www.msaweb.co.uk
Offers information and support to people with MSA, carers and health professionals about multiple system atrophy.

Scottish Disability Sport
Fife Sport Institute
Viewfield Road
Glenrothes KY6 2RB
Tel: 01592 415700
Fax: 01592 415710
Website:
www.scottishdisabilitysport.com
Organizes sports and competition events for people with disabilities. Refers to local branches.

Shirley Price Aromatherapy
Essentia House
Upper Bond Street
Hinckley LE10 1RS
Tel: 01455 615 66
Fax: 01455 615054
Website: www.shirleyprice.com
Sources and supplies natural pure essential oils and carriers for aromatherapy. International college training to professional standards and lists of local therapists accredited by IFPA (International Federation of Professional Aromatherapists) Mail order.

Society of Chiropodists and Podiatrists
1 Fellmongers Path
Tower Bridge Road
London SE1 3LY
Tel: 020 7234 8620
Fax: 020 7234 8621
Website: www.feetforlife.org
Professional association. Provides a guide to foot problems, and help in finding a local chiropodist.

Society of Teachers of the Alexander Technique (STAT)
1st Floor, Linton House
39–51 Highgate Road
London NW5 1RS
Helpline: 0845 230 7828
Tel: 020 7284 3338
Fax: 020 7482 5435
Website: www.stat.org.uk
Offers general information and lists of teachers of the Alexander Technique in the UK and worldwide and recommended training schools. Members receive up-to-date information.

Sport England (previously the Sports Council)
3rd Floor, Victoria House
Bloomsbury Square
London WC1B 4SE
Helpline: 08458 508508
Fax: 020 7383 5740
Website: www.sportengland.org
Government agency promoting sport in England with a wide variety of activity programmes in order to foster a healthier lifestyle.

Sport Scotland (Scottish Sports Council)
Caledonia House
1 Redheughs Rigg
South Gyle
Edinburgh EH12 9DQ
Tel: 0131 317 7200
Fax: 0131 317 7202
Website: www.sportscotland.org.uk
Government agency in Scotland promoting sport with a wide range of activity programmes. Can refer to local sports activities including those for people with disabilities.

Sports Council for Northern Ireland
House of Sport
Upper Malone Road
Belfast BT9 5LA
Tel: 028 9038 1222
Fax: 028 9068 2757
Website: www.sportni.com
Administrative HQ for sport in Northern Ireland with a wide variety of activity programmes catering for able and disabled people; refers to local organizations.

Sports Council for Wales
Sophia Gardens
Cardiff CF11 9SW
Tel: 02920 300500
Fax: 02920 300600
Website:
www.sports-council-wales.co.uk
Headquarters for national network of local clubs who arrange integrated projects to bring disabled and able-bodied people together. Promote sport in Wales and distribute lottery funding. Supports paralympic athletes.

SPRING (Special Parkinson's Research Interest Group)
PO Box 440
Horsham RH13 0YE
Tel: 01403 823947
Website: www.spring.parkinsons.org.uk
Part of Parkinson's Disease Society, this group supports people with a special interest in furthering research into the causes of the disease.

St John Ambulance
27 St John's Lane
London EC1M 4BU
Helpline: 08700 104950
Tel: 08702 355231
Fax: 08700 104065
Website: www.sja.org.uk
Provides first-aid training for
adults and young people and cover
for events. Has a fleet of ambulances
and provides services to homeless
people and library services to
hospitals. Details of local groups
available from HQ or on website.

Tai Chi Northern Ireland
Michele Gibson
22 Station Road
Carnalea
Bangor BT19 1HD
Tel: 028 9146 9400
Fax: 028 9146 9400
Email: taichi.ni@btinternet.com
Representative for Tai Chi Union
offering details of contacts in
Northern Ireland.

Tai Chi Union for Great Britain
1 Littlemill Drive
Balmoral Gardens
Crookston
Glasgow G53 7GF
Tel: 0141 810 3482
Fax: 0141 810 3741
Mobile tel: 07774 985411
Website: www.taichiunion.com
Offers information on different
types of this ancient exercise,
proven to prevent falls in older
people. Can refer to local
instructors or direct to training
courses; SAE required when
requesting information.

Talking Newspapers
Association UK
National Recording Centre
Browning Road
Heathfield TN21 8DB
Tel: 01435 866102
Fax: 01435 865422
Website: www.tnauk.org.uk
Lists 200 national newspapers
and magazines on tape, computer,
CD-ROM and email for loan to
visually impaired, blind and
physically disabled people.
Annual subscription.

Telecottage Association
(Telework Association)
WREN Telecottage
Stoneleigh Park
Kenilworth CV8 2RR
Helpline: 0800 61 60 08
Tel: 02476 696986
Fax: 01453 836174
Website: www.telework.org.uk
Provides information on legal
and practical aspects of setting
up a home business.

THRIVE
Horticultural Therapy
Sir Geoffrey Udall Centre
Beech Hill
Reading RG7 2AT
Tel: 0118 988 5688
Fax: 0118 988 5677
Website: www.thrive.org.uk
Information on gardening and
horticulture for training,
employment, therapy and health.
Uses gardening to help elderly,
disabled or disadvantaged people
to have a better quality of life.

Tremor Foundation
Disablement Services Centre
Harold Wood Hospital (DSC)
Gubbins Lane
Romford RM3 0BE
Helpline: 0800 328 8046
Tel: 01708 386399
Fax: 01708 378032
Website: www.tremor.org.uk
*Volunteers offer support and advice
to people of all ages diagnosed
with any type of tremor. Members
receive regular newsletters and
can attend annual conference with
leading surgeons and neurologists.*

Tripscope
The Vassal Centre
Gill Avenue
Bristol BS16 2QQ
Tel: 08457 585641
Fax: 01179 397736
Minicom 08457 585641
Website: www.tripscope.org.uk
*Provides comprehensive
information for elderly and
disabled people on all aspects of
travelling within the UK and
abroad.*

Ulverscroft Large Print Books
1 The Green
Bradgate Road
Anstey LE7 7FU
Tel: 0116 236 4325
Fax: 0116 234 0205
Website: www.ulverscroft.co.uk
*Publishes large print books,
available at libraries and via
mailorder.*

**United Kingdom Home Care
Association**
42B Banstead Road
Carshalton Beeches SM5 3NW
Tel: 020 8288 1551
Fax: 020 8288 1550
Website: www.ukhca.co.uk
*National representative
association for independent sector
providers of private nursing care
to people in their own homes. Can
supply information and lists of
organizations adhering to
approved code of practice.*

**University of the Third Age
(U3A)**
Third Age Trust
19 East Street
Bromley BR1 1QH
Tel: 020 8466 6139
Fax: 020 8466 5749
Website: www.u3a.org.uk
*Learning cooperative for older
people. Enables members to share
informally many educational,
creative and leisure activities*

**Welsh Sports Association
for the Disabled**
21 Keirhardie Terrace
Softryd
Crymlin
Blaenau NP11 5EJ
Tel: 01495 248861
*Charity offering information on
sports for the disabled. Advises on
suitable sports and refers to local
affiliated clubs.*

Winged Fellowship Trust
Angel House
20–32 Pentonville Road
LondonN1 9XD
Tel: 020 7833 2594
Fax: 020 7278 0370
Website: www.wft.org.uk
Provides holidays at their own UK centres and overseas and respite care for people with severe physical disabilities by providing volunteer carers. Also arranges holidays for people with dementia/Alzheimer's disease and their own carers.

YAPP&Rs
(Young Alert Parkinson's, Partners and Relatives)
YAPMAIL
PO Box 33209
London SW1V 1WH
Helpline: 0808 800 0303
Special interest group of the Parkinson's Disease Society, which supports all young-onset people, families and carers with information, regular meetings and activities. PDS Helpline will put you in touch with the current YAPP&Rs contact.

Yoga for Health Foundation
Ickwell Bury
Biggleswade SG18 9EF
Tel: 01767 627271
Fax: 01767 627266
Website:
www.yogaforhealthfoundation.co.uk
Promotes practice of yoga for all – from the fittest to the most seriously disabled.

Appendix 2
Useful publications

Parkinson's Disease Society publications

Many PDS publications have been mentioned in this book. An up-to-date publications list for people with Parkinson's and their families (B27) is available from the address below. There is also a publications list for professionals (B28). You can also view these publication lists and download most of the general publications and information sheets from the PDS website – www.parkinsons.org.uk

Apart from the videos and one or two other resources, most items are available free except for postage and packing costs. As postage charges are likely to increase from time to time, contact the address below or check the PDS website for current costs. Where a publication has been mentioned in this book that carries a charge, this has been indicated where it appears in the text.

> Sharward Services
> Westerfield Business Centre
> Main Road
> Westerfield
> Ipswich IP6 9AB
> Tel: 01473 212115
> Email: services@sharward.co.uk

Books published elsewhere

These books, unless otherwise indicated, should be available from a bookshop or library. Many books can also be ordered from an Internet-based bookseller such as Amazon (www.amazon.co.uk) or Blackwell's Online Bookshop) (www.blackwells.co.uk). A library can also order books that are not held by them, through interlibrary loans. Quoting the ISBN number listed with each book can help the library or bookshop locate the book. Prices are quoted where known but are subject to change.

General books about Parkinson's

Parkinson's Disease: a self-help guide for patients and their carers, by Dr Marjan Jahanshahi and Professor C. David Marsden, published by Souvenir Press, London (1996) ISBN 0 285 63317 1

The Parkinson's Disease Handbook, by Dr Harvey Sagar, published by Vermillion Press, London (2002) ISBN 0 09 18838 73

100 Questions & Answers about Parkinson's Disease, by Dr Abraham Lieberman with Marcia McCall, published by Jones and Bartlett Publishers, Boston (2003) ISBN 0 7637 0433 4

Books aimed at younger people with Parkinson's

When Parkinson's Strikes Early: voices, choices, resources and treatment, by Barbara Blake-Krebs and Linda Herman, published by Hunter House Publishers, California (2002) ISBN 0 89793 340 0

Books by and about people with Parkinson's

Parkinson's: a patient's view, by Sidney Dorros (British edition with an introduction by Les Essex), Class Publishing, London (1998) ISBN 1 872362 70 2

Health is Between Your Ears: living with a chronic illness, by Svend Andersen. Available from www.parkinsoninfo.dk ISBN 87 88130 49 5

Lucky Man: a memoir, by Michael J. Fox, published by Ebury Press, London (2003) ISBN 0091 885 67 1

Living Well with Parkinson's, by Glenna Wotton Atwood, published by John Wiley & Sons Inc, New Jersey (1991) ISBN 0471 52539 1

Voices from the Parking Lot: Parkinson's insights and perspectives, edited by Dennis Greene, Joan Blessington Snyder, and Craig L Kendall. Available from The Parkinson's Alliance, 211 College Road East, 3rd Floor, Princeton, NJ 08540, USA. Telephone: 001 609 688 0875. Website: www.parkinsonalliance.net

Health issues

How to Get the Most from Your Doctor, by Dr Jonathan Douglas,
    published by Bloomsbury Publishing, London (1993)
    ISBN 0 7475 1292 2
The Patient's Internet Handbook, by Robert Kiley and Elizabeth
    Graham, published by Royal Society of Medicine Press, London
    (2002) ISBN 1 85315 498 9

Practical aspects

*All Dressed Up: a guide to choosing clothes and useful dressing
    techniques for elderly people and people with disabilities*,
    produced by the Disabled Living Foundation, London. See Appendix
    1 for contact details.
The BT Guide for Disabled People, available from British Telecom. See
    Appendix 1 for contact details.
Choosing Eating and Drinking Equipment, published by the Disabled
    Living Foundation. See Appendix 1 for contact details.
Choosing a Telephone, Textphone and Accessories, produced by the
    Disabled Living Foundation. See Appendix 1 for contact details.
Dealing with Someone Else's Money, available from Carers UK. See
    Appendix 1 for contact details.
Escorts and Carers, available from the Holiday Care Service. See
    Appendix 1 for contact details.
*Flying High – a practical guide to air travel for elderly people and
    people with disabilities*, produced by the Disabled Living
    Foundation, London. See Appendix 1 for contact details.
A Garden for You, produced by the Disabled Living Foundation,
    London. See Appendix 1 for contact details.
In Good Repair, published by Care and Repair. See Appendix 1 for
    contact details.
Grow it Yourself: gardening with a physical disability, by Roddy
    Llewellyn and Ann Davies, published by Hutchinson Children's
    Books (1993) ISBN 0749314311
*Historic Houses, Castles and Gardens (incorporating museums &
    galleries)*, published regularly by Conde Nast Johansens Ltd.
    ISBN 1903665000
Hospital Discharge and Continuing Care in England (Factsheet 13),

available from Counsel and Care. See Appendix 1 for contact details.

Information for Visitors with Disabilities, published by the National
Trust, London. See Appendix 1 for contact details.

A Kitchen for You, produced by the Disabled Living Foundation,
London. See Appendix 1 for contact details.

Legal Arrangements for Managing Financial Affairs (Factsheet 22),
available from the Age Concern. See Appendix 1 for contact details.

Making a Complaint about Community Care and NHS Services
(Factsheet 18), available from Counsel and Care. See Appendix 1 for
contact details.

National Gardens Scheme Handbook, available from the National
Gardens Scheme. See Appendix 1 for contact details.

National Trust Handbook, available from the National Trust. See
Appendix 1 for contact details.

Taking a Break, available from Carers UK. See Appendix 1 for contact
details.

The Traveller's Guide To Health, published by the Department of
Health. Available from your local post office or by calling
0800 555777.

What to Look for in a Care Home (Factsheet 19), available from
Counsel and Care. See Appendix 1 for contact details.

Carers

The Carer's Handbook: what to do and who to turn to, by Marina
Lewycka, published by Age Concern England
ISBN 0 86242 262 0

Caring for Someone at a Distance, by Julie Spencer-Cingöz, published
by Age Concern England (2003) ISBN 0 86242 367 8

Caring for Someone with Dementia, by Jane Brotchie, published by
Age Concern England (2003) ISBN 0 86242 368 6

Charities Digest, published by the Family Welfare Association
(updated every year). Your local library should have copies.

Coping with Dementia (Non-professionals can obtain copies from
Alzheimer's Scotland – Action on Dementia. Professionals and
organizations can obtain it from NHS Scotland). See Appendix 1 for
contact details.

A Guide to Grants for Individuals in Need, published by the Directory
of Social Change (updated every year). Your local library should
have copies or see Appendix 1 for contact details.

*Sources of Funding and Obtaining Equipment for Disabled and
Older People*, published by the Disabled Living Foundation. See
Appendix 1 for contact details.

Websites

Listed below are some Parkinson's websites that you may find helpful.
These are given for information purposes only and the publishers of this
book are not responsible for and do not necessarily endorse everything
they contain.

Please note: Websites do not always remain active, and some may
shut down on occasion. Not all websites are reliable. Anyone with some
computer skills can set up a website on any subject. Some may contain
information that is incorrect, or malicious in intention. If you are looking
for factual information on Parkinson's or related subjects, it is important
to check the origin of the websites you are investigating to see whether
the information is anecdotal (i.e. based on someone's individual personal
experience or opinion) or based on reliable scientific fact or research.
Most sites will have an 'about this site' section where you can obtain
more information about the site and who has set it up.

The Canadian Health Network has produced some useful guidelines
for accessing health information on the Internet, to make people aware
of some simple questions that should be asked about the site and
the information it provides. These guidelines can be found at
www.canadian-health-network.ca. If you are concerned about any
information that you come across on the Internet, please discuss it
either with your doctor or another health professional.

- Parkinson's Disease Society – www.parkinsons.org.uk

- SPRING – http://spring.parkinsons.org.uk (The PDS special interest
  group for people interested in medical research.)

- YAPP&Rs – www.youngonset-parkinsons.org.uk (The PDS special
  interest group for younger people of working age with
  Parkinson's and their families.)

- European Parkinson's Disease Association (EPDA) –
  www.epda.eu.com (Provides information about EPDA activities and
  links to member organizations.)

- *Awakenings – Parkinson's Disease* – www.parkinsonsdisease.com
  (Lifestyle-management advice, a glossary of terms, treatment
  options and a book list. Features drug information and
  support-group details.)

- National Parkinson Foundation (Florida, USA) – www.parkinson.org
  (Latest news and developments in Parkinson's disease research.
  Includes a list of publications and events, and an 'Ask the Doctor'
  facility which you can subscribe to.)

- Parkinson's Disease Foundation (New York, USA) – www.pdf.org
  (Up-to-date news, an 'Ask the Expert' facility, and a free on-line
  newsletter.)

- American Parkinson Disease Association (New York, USA)
  www.apdaparkinson.com (Booklets available for free download,
  and a section for people with young-onset Parkinson's.)

- Parkinson's Web (USA) – http://pdweb.mgh.harvard.edu
  (Comprehensive data and listings on Parkinson's. Includes
  support and treatment resources.)

- Michael J Fox Foundation – www.michaeljfox.org (An organization,
  set up by Michael J Fox, dedicated to fundraising and
  sponsorship of research into Parkinson's.)

- Chris Chapman – www.young-parkinsons.org.uk (Chris Chapman is
  a young man with Parkinson's living in the UK. This website gives
  his personal account of living with Parkinson's.)

- P-I-E-N – www.parkinsons-information-exchange-network-online.com
  (An international Internet discussion group for younger people
  with Parkinson's.)

- Parkinson's Association of Ireland – http://gofree.indigo.ie/~pdpals/
  (PALS is the Parkinson's Association of Ireland's group for
  younger people with Parkinson's. This website contains
  information and personal pieces by young people living with
  Parkinson's in Ireland.)

Parkinson's
Disease Society

Parkinson's Disease Society of the United Kingdom

The Society's mission is: The conquest of Parkinson's disease and the alleviation of the distress it causes, through effective research, welfare, education and communication.

For help and advice about Parkinson's, please contact the PDS Helpline at the phone number given below.

☐ Please send me the introductory booklet about Parkinson's disease and the Parkinson's Disease Society (includes a membership form).

☐ Please send me details of the PDS special interest group for younger people with Parkinson's (YAPP&Rs).

☐ Please send me details of the PDS special interest group for research (SPRING).

☐ I am a professional working with people with Parkinson's. Please send me your professionals publications list.

An A5 SAE with stamps to the value of 58p would be appreciated.

The PDS always needs donations and practical help to carry on its work. Could you help?

☐ I would like to volunteer.

☐ Please send me a Gift Aid Declaration form.

☐ Please send me information on making a will and leaving a legacy.

☐ Please send me fundraising information.

☐ I enclose a donation of £_____ (made payable to the Parkinson's Disease Society). For credit card donations call 020 7932 1349.

Name: _____

Address: _____

_____

Postcode: _____ Telephone: _____

Please return this form to: The Parkinson's Disease Society, 215 Vauxhall Bridge Road, London SW1V 1EJ. Telephone: 020 7931 8080. Website: www.parkinsons.org.uk Helpline: 0808 800 0303 Textphone (Minicom): 020 7963 9380 Email enquiries: enquiries@parkinsons.org.uk

Parkinson's Disease Society of the United Kingdom. Registered charity number: 258197. A company limited by guarantee. Registered No. 948776 (London). Registered Office: 215 Vauxhall Bridge Road, London SW1V 1EJ.

Index